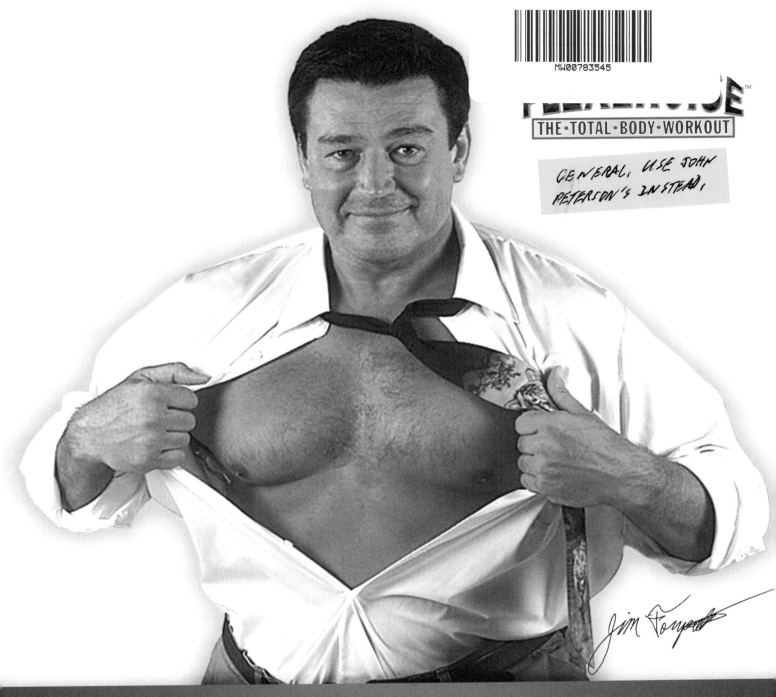

THE·TOTAL·BODY·WORKOUT

GENERAL, USE JOHN
PETERSON'S INSTEAD,

POWeRFLEX
UNLEASH the POWER in YOU!
by Jim Forystek

BRONZE BOW PUBLISHING

POWERFLEX

by Flexercise™
Copyright © 1997, 2005 Jim Forystek

Flexercise™ is a trademark that is the exclusive property of Jim Forystek.

ISBN 1-932458-25-5

Published by Bronze Bow Publishing Inc.,
2600 E. 26th Street, Minneapolis, MN 55406.

You can reach us on the Internet at www.bronzebowpublishing.com

Literary development and cover/interior design by
Koechel Peterson & Associates, Inc., Minneapolis, Minnesota.

Manufactured in the United States of America

TABLE OF CONTENTS

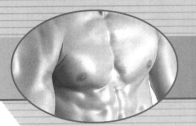

4	Acknowledgments
8	Foreword
10	Preface
11	Introduction
13	Welcome to the Wild World of Flexercise™
17	Chest Workout
33	Abdominal Workout
49	Spine Workout
65	Neck Workout
81	Back Workout
96	Taking Stock
97	Leg Workout
113	Shoulder Workout
129	Arm Workout
145	Speed, Energy, and Endurance Workout
153	A Final Word
154	Question & Answers

ACKNOWLEDGMENTS

When I first published my Flexercise™ program in 1997, I had already used it to train several championship teams and individuals in a variety of sports. At that time, my sons, Jimmy (age 11) and Johnny (age 9), were eager to build their muscles and excel in sports. They began to train using the Flexercise™ exercises exclusively—no weights, pulleys, machines, or pills. The rippling muscles, athletic endurance, and physiques they gained were awesome, just as this program had worked for me. They loved the results and began to excel beyond their wildest imaginations.

By the time they were 15 and 17 years old, respectively, they entered a national bodybuilding competition (one in which everyone knew substance enhancement was being used). The boys wanted to prove that an all-natural Flexercise™ person could stand out without using steroids, drugs, pills, or illegal substances. Not surprising to me, they blew the crowd away with their routines! I can still hear the screams and cheers! Both Jimmy and Johnny came home with huge trophies!

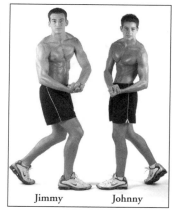

Jimmy   Johnny

Both boys have continued doing Flexercise™, and they are the two models along with me in this book. Jimmy now plays college football for the Liberty Flames, an NCAA Division 1 team in Virginia. The Flames' new strength coach came from the Seattle Seahawks and put the entire team through a strength and endurance test he didn't expect anyone to pass. Out of 63 players, Jimmy was one of only three players who made it through the test, and he did it as a freshman!

Johnny continues to blow away the high school record book whenever it comes to the strength, push-ups, and sit-ups testing. For their obstacle course testing, he ran it while carrying another student piggyback and finished ahead of most of the other runners. Being fit and having the body you want is such a source of joy and personal satisfaction.

I would like to thank the people who have encouraged me to be fit and strong, starting with my grandfather, Lawrence Blindauer, who served in World War I under General Pershing. "Pup," as we called him, always exercised and taught me how important exercise is for the body. He showed me many exercises they did to be strong for battle and proved you don't need weights or special machines to do it. He lived to be 88 years old, stayed in his own home, and had just passed his driver's license renewal before he went home to glory.

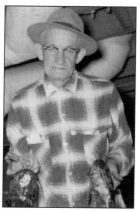

I want to thank my dad, Thaddeus, better known as "Ted," who served in World War II under General Patton and chased the infamous "Desert Fox," General Rommel, through the deserts of Africa. He never lifted weights or used machines or equipment, but he is undoubtedly the strongest man I have ever known. He exercised but used his own body's energy and ability alone. He amazed my brothers and me whenever we went with him to help move someone. In the time it took us to get the couch off the back of the truck and into the house, my dad would have the refrigerator, the washer, and the dryer off the back of the truck all by himself!

I will never forget an experience that forever showed me my dad's inner and outer strength. He had taken two of my sisters, my niece, my brother Sam, and me to the northern Wisconsin woods to pick blackberries. As kids, we would gather just enough berries to satisfy our tastes and then play in the woods until my dad filled all our pails. On this trip, Sam and I spotted a tall tree slightly leaning to the side and wondered if we could push it over. As our sisters and niece watched nearby, we rocked the tree back and forth until finally it cracked and hit the ground with a thud and split open.

We didn't know that inside the tree was a gigantic bees' nest that also split wide open, and instantly we were all being stung by hundreds of angry swarming bees. Our screams were loud! Bees were everywhere. We tried swatting them out of one another's hair and off backs and arms, then we all ran for the car, hollering all the way. In a woods where it's common to come upon huge bears, trophy bucks, and wild bobcats, you can imagine what my father thought was happening to us!

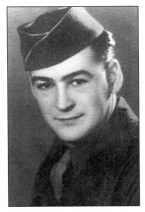

My father came running faster than I ever believed he could move, and in his hands he carried a six-foot long solid metal pipe just as a pole-vaulter does, which he was ready to ram through the heart of any creature that was attacking us. He thought we were being mauled by a bear, of course, and was relieved to see it was only bees! Somewhere in those woods there was a very lucky bear. Only God knows what would have happened to that mighty critter if my dad had come upon it before he knew the situation! Needless to say, Sam and I were in hot water for a long time. Our sisters and niece had to go to the doctor and take medicine to counteract the massive number of stings.

Throughout my life it has been a real comfort and strength to know my dad loved me so much that he was willing to lay down his life to save me. This really came home to roost when I met Jesus Christ by faith after a Billy Graham Crusade and learned this verse from the Good Book: *Greater love hath no man than this, that a man lay down his life for his friends.* I now have two daddies who loved me enough to die for me, and One actually did! We never figured out where my dad found a solid six-foot metal pole in the middle of the woods, but after the trouble we had caused, we never mustered up enough courage to ask him!

My father lived well into his 80s in his own home, and it was fitting that he went home to glory wearing his Mickey Mouse T-shirt from Disneyland and a pair of boxers!

I want to also thank Charles Atlas who carried the natural exercise fitness torch and was a *real inspiration* to me, especially during my teens. Although as a kid I couldn't afford his entire course, he reinforced in me the examples given by my grandfather and dad on the natural way to exercise. Combining and performing all these different techniques since the ninth grade really made an astounding difference in my life. Thank you, Mr. Charles Atlas, or should I say, Mr. Angelo Siciliano?

I *especially* thank my new friend, Mr. John Peterson, President of Bronze Bow Publishing. To say he's one in a million would be too common. I'd say he's more like *one in a billion.* John is a genuine human being. He's open, honest, inspiring, and lights the fire from the inside out. He has a quality that has all but disappeared from this planet, and it's called "integrity." He is also one of the fittest and strongest men I know! His books, *Pushing Yourself to Power* and *The Miracle Seven*, are fantastic, and more proof that you can get the body of your dreams without weights, special machines, or illegal substances. To this day, I do not know what's more powerful—*a keg of dynamite* or *Mr. John Peterson!*

How I met John is very unique. Some time ago I noticed a sharp incline in my Flexercise™ sales and couldn't figure out why. Then a man from England ordered Flexercise™ and asked if I knew John Peterson, who had recommended my book

to him. I had never heard of John, but I came to find out it was because of John that the sales were rising. I found John's phone number and called to thank him. John already had his own excellent workout books for sale, yet he had a big enough heart and enough confidence in himself to recommend my book! Do you know how solid, how full of integrity a person has to be to do that! My friend, it's unheard of! Mr. John Peterson is one of a kind. Thank you, John!

I want to thank the Creator of the animals, such as the panther, eagle, bear, gorilla, and elk, for their natural beauty and raw amazing strength. They are the true inspiration for Flexercise™ and the backbone of the Total Body Workout.

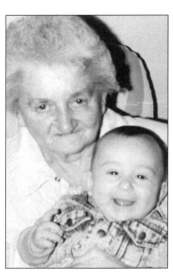

And a special thanks to my mom, Geraldine, who for the health of her children got us off the processed, bleached, and chemical-filled foods and turned us on to whole wheat, whole grain, and honey instead of white sugar. Never forget that "Mom" turned right side up spells "Wow"! God rest her soul.

MISSION STATEMENT

Flexercise™ is dedicated to empowering each person to build the body he or she desires—whether that body is massively muscled like a bull elk, or lean, scultped, and explosive like a panther. Flexercise™ is dedicated to empowering people to build strength, health, and fitness naturally by using their body's own energies and abilities—as the creatures of the animal kingdom do.

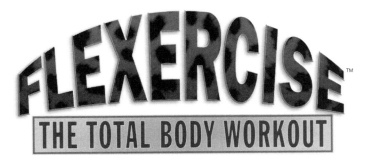

2600 East 26th Street
Minneapolis, MN 55406

flexworkout@aol.com
www.flexerciseworkout.com

FOREWORD *by* JOHN e. PETERSON

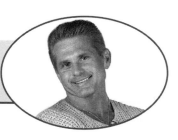

I n early December 2004, I received a phone call at the office. Our receptionist, Bridget, told me that a gentleman by the name of Jim Forystek wanted to speak with me.

Hearing his name, I smiled, picked up the phone, and said, "Big Jim Forystek, this is John Peterson, and I want you to know that it's an honor to speak with you."

There was a long pause on Jim's end, then he finally said, "John, the honor is mine. My Flexercise™ Courses have been practically flying out of here lately, and almost every time I ask someone, 'Where did you hear about my course?' I've been told that John Peterson of Bronze Bow Publishing recommended it to them. Matter of fact, they say that you recommend this as the one course above all others for anyone interested in developing a beautiful physique without having to rely on weights or equipment. And they tell me that 'If Peterson is willing to say that, then I want to buy it.' "

At that point, we both broke out laughing.

"John," Jim continued, "based on your recommendation alone I've even sold one of my Flexercise™ Courses to a man in England. But I'm curious. You've written and published your own book, *Pushing Yourself to Power.* So why do you recommend my course so strongly?"

"Jim," I answered, "I'm not trying to push my religious faith on you, but the truth is that I'm a born-again, Bible-believing Christian, and my mom and dad taught me to tell the truth. And in this case, the truth is simple. Your Flexercise™ Course is the only course I've seen that promotes the same type of health, strength, and physique building exercise that I promote. It doesn't cause 'Busted-Up Weightlifter's Syndrome,' and it doesn't destroy one's joints, tendons, and ligaments in the process or compress and damage the lower spine. In fact, your Flexercise™ Course and my Transformetrics™ Training System in *Pushing Yourself to Power* are like two sides of the same coin. So it's only natural that I'd endorse your course. How could I not?"

At that, Big Jim paused and told me that he too was a born-again, Bible-believing Christian, and that he and his entire family had dedicated themselves to bringing health, strength, and dynamic physical fitness to God's people.

It wasn't long after our phone conversation until Jim drove to our office in Minneapolis, and we determined to work together in providing the people of America with the best, safest, and most effective methods of exercise and physical culture known to man. This book represents our first collaboration together, and I'm excited to publish it under Bronze Bow Publishing.

In the pages that follow, you will be introduced to Big Jim Forystek and his sons, Jimmy and Johnny, who posed for each of the exercise photos throughout the *PowerFlex* training methods. I know you'll agree that these young men, who have used this course since they were young, personify the term "Greek-god physique."

It is our hope that *PowerFlex* will take our readers to a whole new level of lifetime health, strength, and physical fitness. And that it adds years to your life and, even more important, life to your years.

May God bless you richly in health and abundant living,

John E. Peterson

P.S. Wait will you see the *PowerFlex* DVD—awesome stuff! And that's only the beginning.

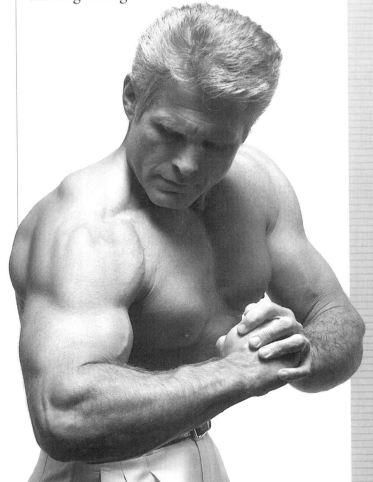

PREFACE

Humans have always depended on animals for food, clothing, shelter, and transportation. Seeing and feeling this dependence inspired men and women to give thanks to the animals whose lives they took to satisfy their needs. Before hunting expeditions, hunters and their extended families would celebrate the strength and courage of their prey in rituals, hoping to inspire the hunters with that same strength and courage.

As civilization developed, humans continued to feel and express not only their dependence on animals, but their kinship with them. When healers in ancient China created qi gong (chee gong), an elaborate system for aligning the body and mind, they created the Five Animal Frolics, five sets of dance-like movements inspired by animals whose qualities they admired.

This book is an original expression of these same feelings and desires.

Flexercise™ is based on the idea that imitating the movements of animals is a simple but powerful route to physical health and wellness. Through careful study of animals and their movements, Jim Forystek has evolved a series of 45 simple Flexercises that require no equipment but the body itself.

Unlike weightlifting, aerobics, and other popular forms of exercise, Flexercise™ strengthens and shapes the body safely, without stressing the joints, connective tissues, and spine. Resistance is determined not by the plates on the bar or the setting on the machine, but by the Flexercisers own ability and desire to maintain tension in the muscles as they work. Thus, Flexercise™ not only develops strength, power, and endurance, but develops the ability to express these qualities through harmonious movement and with athletic grace.

I am very thankful to Jim Forystek, Creator of Flexercise™, and to John Peterson, Founder of Bronze Bow Publishing, for the opportunity to assist in preparing the manuscript of this edition. Considering the frustrations and injuries weightlifting and other popular exercise methods have caused me, I feel fortunate to have had this opportunity to promote such a safe, effective, health-giving one.

As humans rely more and more on technology to run our lives for us, we often feel distant from the natural rhythms of life on earth, and from the animals that share our dependency. May Flexercise™ deepen your appreciation for the animals whose traits and abilities we celebrate here and for the wonder of your own body. Flexercise™ help you enjoy a lifetime of vibrant good health.

Gregg Heinrichs

INTRODUCTION

Welcome to the wonderful world of Flexercise™. I commend you for having the courage to take the step that your body will reward you for an entire lifetime. It is always a great pleasure to know there are people such as you, who take control of their lives and health and go forward with confidence.

Flexercise™ is the most revolutionary and powerful way to exercise for accelerated, powerful, eye-popping results. Yet the principle behind Flexercise™ is so simple. It is so simple and powerful, in fact, that mankind has overlooked it for centuries.

The most powerful, graceful, awe-inspiring, perfectly sculpted specimens of strength and beauty—the ones most appealing to the eyes and most inspiring to the imagination—aren't human beings, but animals. You see it clearly in the off-the-charts strength, exquisite grace, and royal beauty of the lion, which the Bible calls the strongest of beasts. It is also evident in the mesmerizing muscles and agility of the majestic elk that freely roams the upper elevations of the mountains as though child's play despite weighing over 1,000 pounds.

Yet when you consider the pillars of strength, the flexibility, the incredible speed, the ripped muscles, and the beauty of creatures among the animal kingdom, you'll notice there is no workout gym, no special equipment, no weights, no rowing machines, or dumbbells. It is all attained by using their body weight and energy and natural abilities.

It is this same principle that Flexercise™ is built upon, and make not mistake, it works—no ifs and buts. It's not up for questions or debate. The animals have already proven the point a million times, and it worked for me.

Based upon my physique alone, I was offered a full scholarship by the chancellor of a major East Coast college that turns out many professional football players. My chest muscles and upper body strength and overall look was gained through the Flexercise™ program, and the college chancellor was impressed. He wanted me on a plane within two days if I would be the fullback of their team.

I turned down the gracious offer, to pursue my father's business, and I've turned down other offers since then. I've also coached and quarterbacked my own city league team to five championships and raised it to be one of the most feared and respected teams in the league. Because of Flexercise™ and the energy and glow and respectability it has given me as a person, I've grown accustomed to the notices, advances, and opportunities that come my way that others dream about.

Wherever I am, I am constantly approached and have doors opened for me by people who mistake me for a professional football player, an Olympic weightlifter, a bodybuilder, a professional wrestler, or an actor. My physique gets their attention, and they think that I must be someone special. Countless people have approached me and asked how many hours I spend in the gym a day, how much I bench press, and how I attained this level of physical fitness. Knowing that a proud arrogant braggart is the most unattractive person in the world, I usually respond to their inquiries by saying, "I'm on the George Foreman workout program—McDonalds for breakfast and Burger King for lunch."

Seriously, though, after you've sculpted your muscles, please feel free to tell your admirers that it's due to Flexercise™.

Now let's get to it!

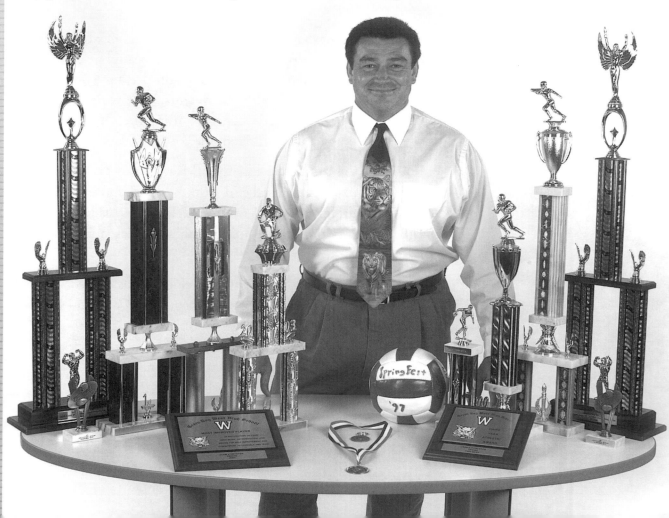

Welcome to the Wild
WORLD OF FLEXERCISE™

Thank you for choosing Flexercise™, the total body workout program. Make no mistake: Flexercise™ gives real results that you will be pleased with, and results without the use of steroids, drugs, weights, or expensive workout equipment. This program is based upon the same principles that build the most awesome, powerful, beautiful bodies of some species within the animal kingdom.

Still, you don't need to be as powerful as the gorilla or as fast as the panther to benefit from this course. The beauty of Flexercise™ is that it lets you start where you are, at your current level of fitness, and you can use it to reach your fitness goals, whatever they are. If you want huge, bulging muscles like a bull elk, put high tension and muscle resistance into each movement while performing your Flexercises. But if your goal is to be toned and sleek like a panther, with healthy muscle definition and shape, ease up on the level of resistance you put into each movement and exercise. You can develop your body the way you want it to be!

Workout Rotation

To get started with Flexercise™, I recommend that you rotate the sets of exercises that concentrate on different muscle groups in this fashion:

> **Week 1:** Chest Workout only
> **Week 2:** Chest and Abdominal Workouts
> **Week 3:** Chest, Spine, and Neck Workouts
> **Week 4:** Chest and Back Workouts
> **Week 5:** Chest and Leg Workouts
> **Week 6:** Chest and Shoulder Workouts
> **Week 7:** Chest and Arm Workouts
> **Week 8:** Chest and Speed, Energy, and Endurance Workouts

It's important for you to do the Chest Workout for all eight weeks of this course. This is because the Flexercises in the Chest Workout will force you to breathe deeply, which will trigger muscle growth and development throughout your body.

Once you've completed the entire course, you can repeat the cycle again, if you wish. Or you can replace the Chest Workout with one of the other Workouts, rotating the other Workouts weekly for eight weeks until you've done them all.

Another option is to build your own routine by choosing one exercise from each Workout. Since each of the Workouts in this course contains five Flexercises, you have a wide variety to choose from to prevent boredom as you continue to develop your body.

Building your own routine allows you to focus on problem areas. For example, if you want to focus on your abdominals, do the whole Abdominal Workout during every session, along with at least one Flexercise™ from each of the other Workouts. Your routine would look like this:

Dolphin Flex I
Dolphin Flex II
Shark Flex I
Shark Flex II
Dolphin Flex III
A Chest Exercise
A Spine Exercise
A Neck Exercise
A Back Exercise
A Leg Exercise
A Shoulder Exercise
An Arm Exercise
A Speed, Energy, and Endurance Exercise

Follow this routine for as long you want, then pick another area to focus on and begin again.

The sky's the limit, and it's your body to transform—get creative and use Flexercise™ to your best advantage to build the body you desire!

Number of Repetitions

Along with instructions for performing each Flexercise™ in this course, I've listed a recommended number of repetitions to do, based on how advanced a Flexerciser is. Level One is for beginners; Level Two is for intermediate trainees, and Level Three is for advanced trainees.

Whether you're new to regular exercise or are already fit from other activities, you shouldn't go beyond Level One during your first week of training. If you can't do the number of repetitions listed for Level One, that's fine—begin your journey where you are. Even if you're already fit, you won't have to go beyond Level One to get an excellent workout at this stage. That's because, with Flexercise™, *the key to success isn't the number of repetitions you do: it's the amount of tension you use.*

As you do each Flexercise™, concentrate on the muscles that particular Flexercise™ is designed to work, and try to maintain constant tension in those muscles. Use enough tension so that you perform each Flexercise™ slowly, but not so much tension that you're uncomfortable—train, don't strain! Try to breathe through your nose, not your mouth. If you find yourself panting, back off the tension immediately. Never hold your breath!

When you can do your repetitions while maintaining constant tension in the working muscles and without straining, add one more repetition to that Flexercise™ the next time you do it. Don't add another repetition for that exercise for at least a week. This will give your body time to adapt to the new workload and will help you avoid over-training.

It's a good idea to log your workouts in a notebook. Writing down the Flexercises and the number of repetitions you do gives you a record of your progress.

Building the Mind-Muscle Connection

I can't emphasize enough that your ability to develop the body you want will depend less on the number of repetitions you do than on the amount of tension you use while doing them. This is a subject I've discussed at length with my good friend John Peterson, who stresses this point in two excellent books teaching the Transformetrics™ Training System he created. Learning to apply just enough tension to maximize growth—to build the connection between your mind and muscles—is a skill that consistent, patient practice of Flexercise™ will allow you to master.

Building the mind-muscle connection isn't as tough as it sounds, provided you do two things: perform your Flexercises in front of a full-length mirror and wear clothing that lets you see your muscles working. Watching yourself while Flexercising will help you use

proper technique and will show you how different amounts of tension affect how your muscles look—the more tense your biceps muscle is, for example, the bigger your upper arm will appear in the mirror.

As you do each Flexercise™, try to "think into" the muscle that's working. For example, as you do Gorilla Flex IV

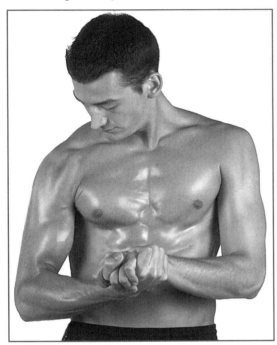

(the first biceps Flexercise™ in the Arm Workout), focus your eyes on your biceps as your arm flexes and extends. Imagine the way you want your biceps to look. Improving your mind-muscle connection through Flexercise™ will improve your ability to use the strength you're developing, whether you're sweeping the kitchen floor, changing a flat tire, or throwing a touchdown pass—and move with the purpose, agility, and grace of a wild animal.

Workout Frequency

Some people do two or three Flexercise™ sessions per week. But if you want to see quick improvement, I recommend working out at least five times per week.

Flexercises can be done anywhere, anytime, and don't require special equipment. You could even Flexercise™ five times per week while watching your favorite half-hour TV show and finish your workout before the show ends!

Whether you work out five, three, or two days per week, what matters most is that you're consistent, week in and week out. Stick with it and don't quit! No excuses! Your body will thank you for it a million times over!

Now get at it!

DON'T QUIT

When things go wrong, as they sometimes will,
When the road you're trudging seems all uphill,
When the funds are low, and the debts are high,
And you want to smile, but you have to sigh,
When care is pressing you down a bit,
Rest if you must, but never quit.

Life is strange, with its twists and turns,
As everyone of us sometimes learns,
And many a failure turns about
When he might have won, had he stuck it out.

Don't give up, though the pace seems slow:
You may succeed with another blow.
Success is a failure turned inside out,
The silver lining in the cloud of doubt.

And you can never tell how close you are.
It may be nearer, when it seems so far.
So stick to the fight when you're the hardest hit.
It's when things seem worst that you must not quit.

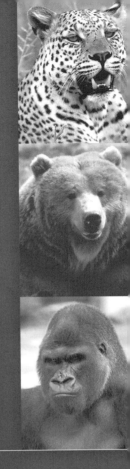

POWERFLEX
CHEST

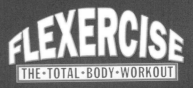

CHEST WORKOUT

The Flexercise™ program for building a huge, powerful, massive chest, without special equipment or steroids, is based on the principle of five of the most powerful animals that possess massive chest strength—the panther, eagle, bear, gorilla, and elk. All you need are five simple Flexercises, 20 minutes per day, and your own best effort!

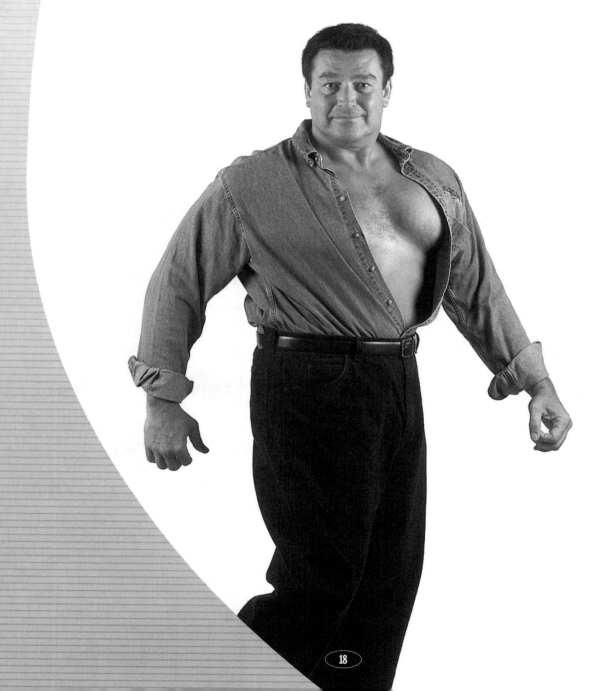

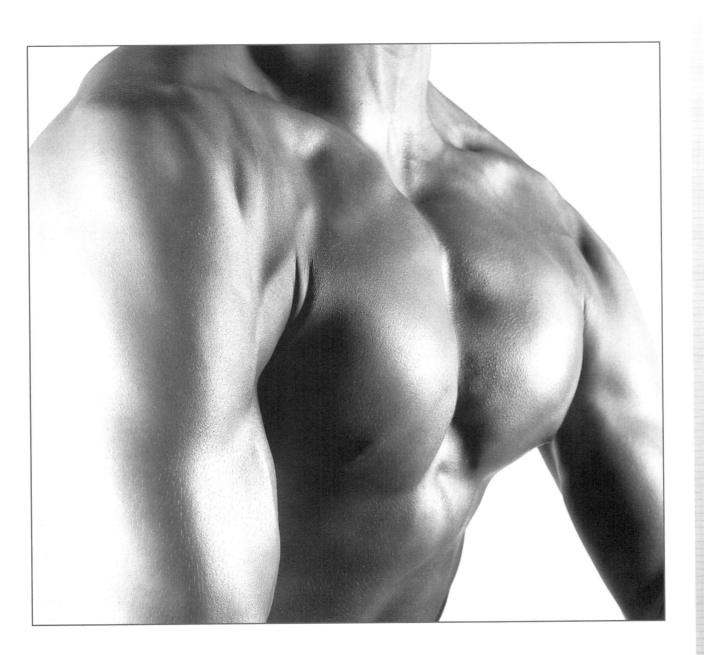

#1 PANTHER FLEX I

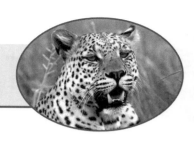

You'll notice when a panther or any member of the cat family gets ready to strike their prey, they crouch and flex their massive chest muscles that give them such extraordinary leaping ability as they spring upon their mark. The Panther Flex stimulates that flex for the chest. We've all done push-ups from time to time—well now get ready to take the humble push-up to the next level.

To do the Panther Flex, do push-ups between two chairs (or any sturdy objects of equal height). Set your chairs just a little wider than shoulder-width apart and let your body sink a little lower than the chairs as you go down. It's this extra flex that feeds and nourishes and works your chest muscles with staggering results. Don't be fooled, this Flexercise™ will give you what you're looking for. It's for real.

> **LEVEL THREE:** 100 repetitions
> **LEVEL TWO:** 40 repetitions
> **LEVEL ONE:** 20 repetitions

REMEMBER: If your goal is to develop a massive, imposing physique, you'll need to use more tension while doing your Flexercises than someone whose goal is to develop a lean, more defined physique.

Sometimes I do 100 repetitions all at once, and other times I break up those repetitions into sets, resting a bit between each set (70 + 30, or 50 + 50, or 30 + 40 + 30, etc.). Feel free to break up your repetitions into sets, too. Experiment to see what works for you and don't do more than you're comfortable with.

What matters most is that you do your Flexercises consistently—day after day, week after week, month after month. You won't have long to wait, though, before your consistency and patience start to reap their rewards.

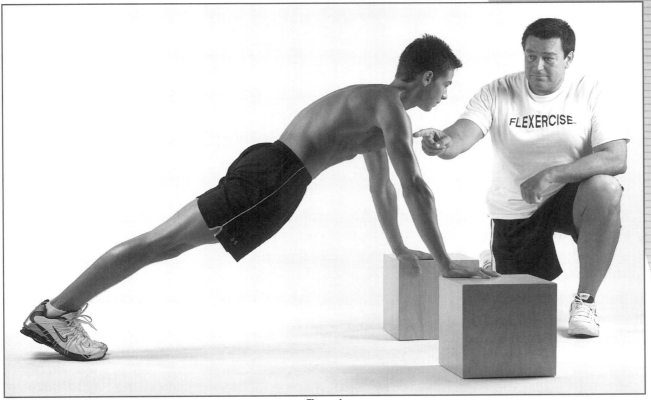

Figure 1

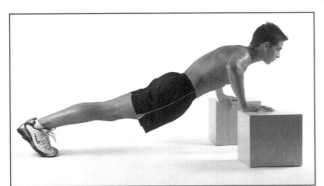

Figure 2

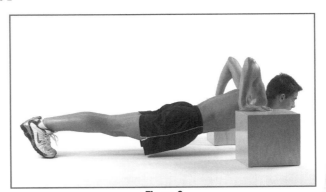

Figure 3

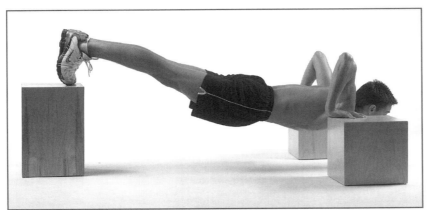

ADVANCED

#2 EAGLE FLEX I

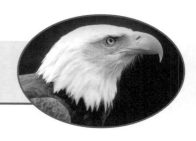

It's no wonder that the eagle is the symbol of the greatest country on earth. Its broad wings carry it to great heights—even above mountaintops. The eagle owes this ability to its incredible chest muscles, which flex each time it flaps its wings.

To perform the Eagle Flex, stand straight up with your feet shoulder-width apart and your arms straight down at your sides. With fingers extending with an open hand, slowly raise your arms, keeping them straight as an eagle's wing, while flexing your chest muscles. Reach and extend farther as you raise your arms and extend them as wings. Extend them until your hands are just a little higher than your head, then bring your arms down slightly in front of you, now flexing your chest muscles on the way down, until your hands cross in front of you. Breathe in as you go up—fill your lungs—and exhale as you come down. Reverse the movement and repeat.

This exercise develops the chest muscles quickly, and the deep breathing it involves will stimulate muscle growth throughout your body.

LEVEL THREE: 60 repetitions
LEVEL TWO: 30 repetitions
LEVEL ONE: 15 repetitions

CHEST

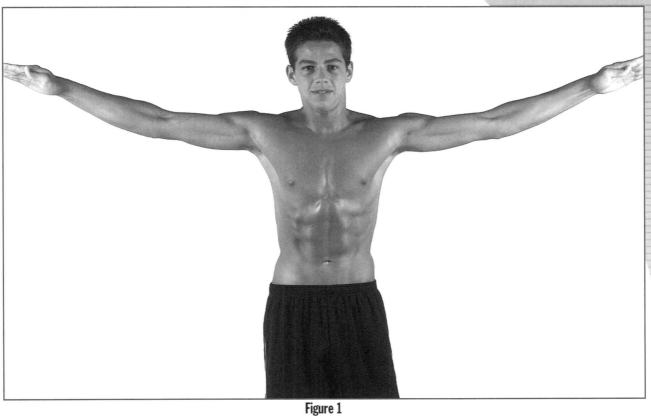

Figure 1

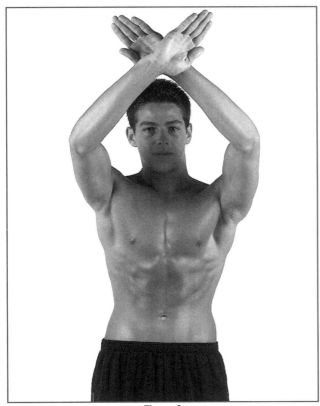

Figure 2

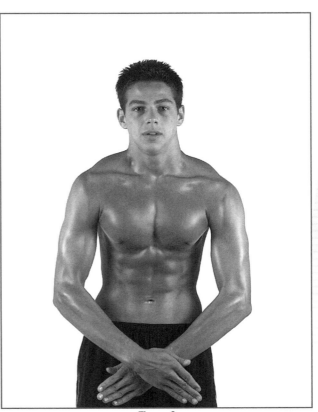

Figure 3

#3 BEAR FLEX I

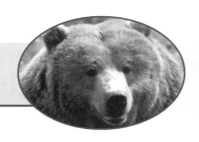

There's only one way to describe the embrace that can take your breath away and crush your bones: the bear hug. The bear is admired and feared for its ability to crush the life out of creatures. The Bear Flex I simulates a bear hug.

Stand with your hands in front of you, a little lower than your waist. With one hand turned up and the other turned down, grip and interlock your fingers in a cupped position. With your fingers locked and pulling apart, slowly lift your hands while keeping them close to your body until your hands are over your head, flexing your chest muscles as you do it. Keep the tension on, pulling apart with fingers interlocked. Then slowly move back down to the starting position.

LEVEL THREE: 40 repetitions
LEVEL TWO: 25 repetitions
LEVEL ONE: 10 repetitions

CHEST

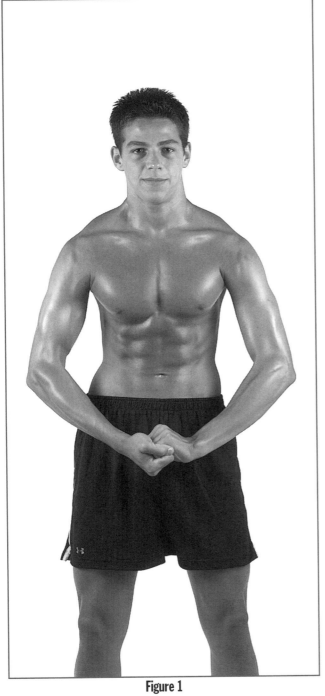

Figure 1

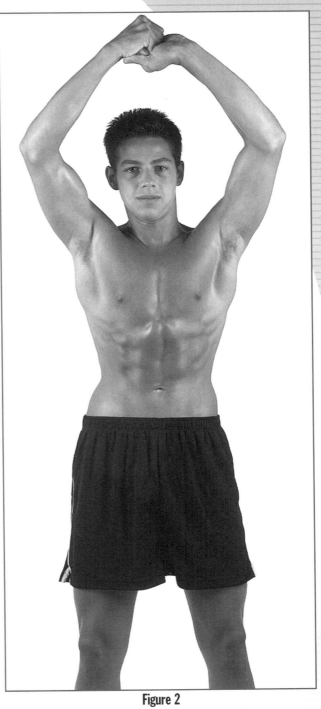

Figure 2

#4 GORILLA FLEX I

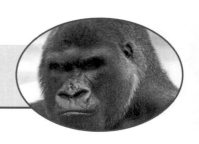

The massive gorilla pounds proudly on his immense chest to display his superiority. Considering their size, gorillas display mind-boggling strength and agility through their swinging and climbing on vines and branches. Fortunately, you don't need vines, branches, or special equipment to simulate this movement, thanks to the Gorilla Flex I.

Imagine there's a climbing rope hanging in front of you. Standing with your feet shoulder-width apart, grab that imaginary rope, clinch it in your fists lightly in front of you just above your head. Then flex your chest muscles as you slowly pull that rope down. Flex, pull, and grip with each hand, alternately, until both hands are a bit lower than your waist. Raise your hands above your head again and repeat.

LEVEL THREE: 40 repetitions
LEVEL TWO: 20 repetitions
LEVEL ONE: 10 repetitions

CHEST

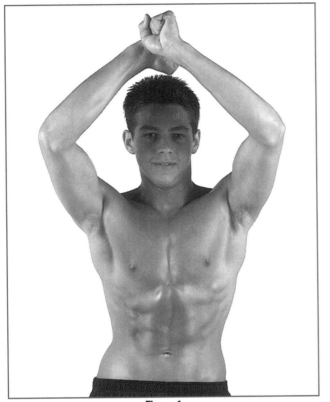

Figure 1

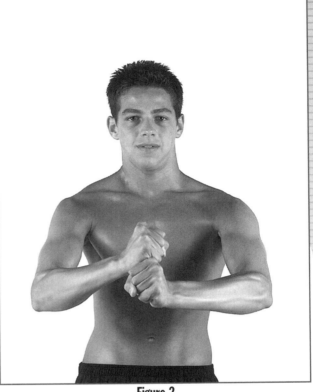

Figure 2

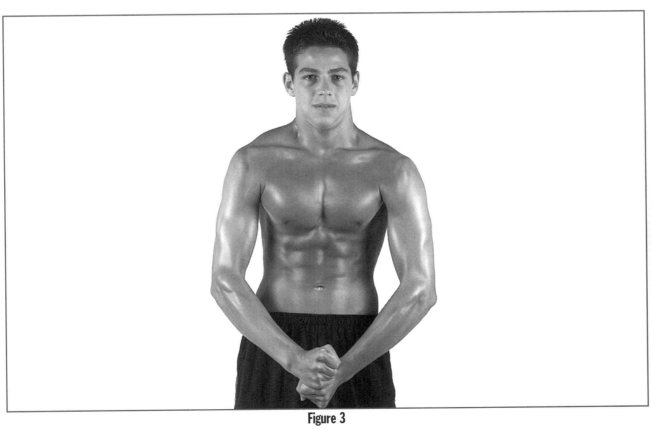

Figure 3

#5 BULL ELK FLEX I

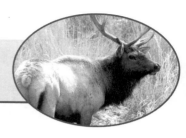

One glimpse of a bull elk in the wild is enough to make the strongest heart feel faint! Its massive chest contains the powerful lungs that allow it to climb mountaintops at over 10,000 feet with ease. The Bull Elk Flex I brings into play the working of the elk's chest as he flexes his chest against the resistance of climbing the mountain.

Make a fist with one hand and place the fist in the palm of the other hand, with your knuckles on the palm and the inside of the fisted hand close to your body. Keep your upper arms straight at your sides, slightly ahead of you, bending only at the elbows. Start with the palm of the hand about chest high, then push down on that palm with your fist, resisting the fist with the palm and flexing your chest muscles, just as a bull elk goes up a mountainside. Slowly allow the fist to overcome the palm, forcing the arm down slowly until it is a little lower than your waist. Now do the same exercise on the other side, reversing the position of your hands.

LEVEL THREE: 40 repetitions (20 per side)
LEVEL TWO: 20 repetitions
LEVEL ONE: 10 repetitions

Performing these five Flexercises with consistency, determination, and patience will earn you the chest development you desire—all without steroids, special equipment, or even a gym membership. It won't be long before you see the fruit of your labors. Please feel free to call, write, or email me and let me know how you're progressing. I want to rejoice in your progress with you!

However far along you are with Flexercise™, I want to commend you again for your determination to improve your fitness, appearance, and health—to "walk the walk," not just "talk the talk"!

CHEST

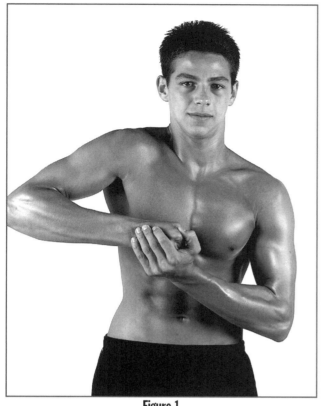

Figure 1

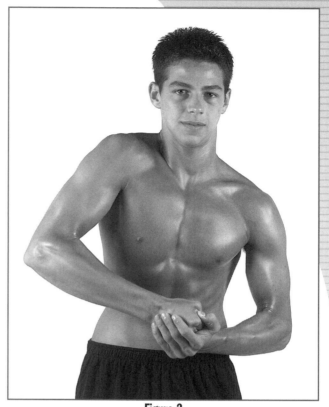

Figure 2

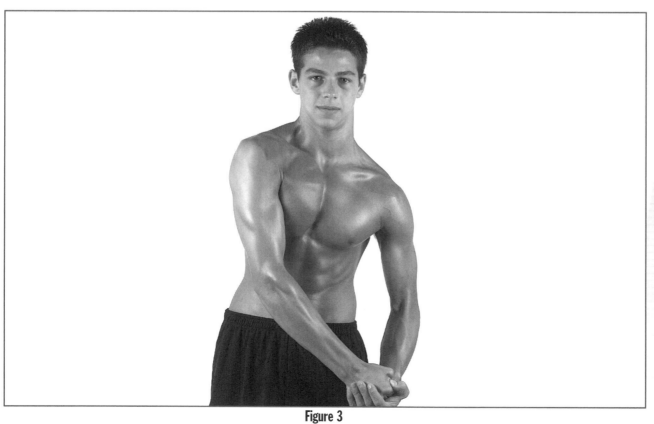

Figure 3

POWERFLEX

CHEST EXERCISES

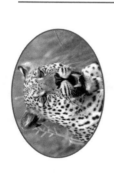

PANTHER FLEX | figure 1

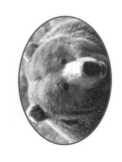

EAGLE FLEX | figure 2

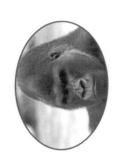

BEAR FLEX | figure 3

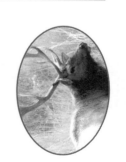

GORILLA FLEX | figure 4

ELK FLEX | figure 5

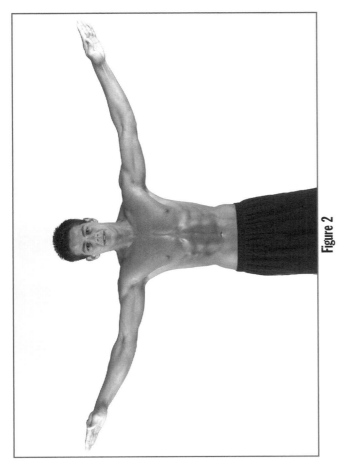

Figure 2

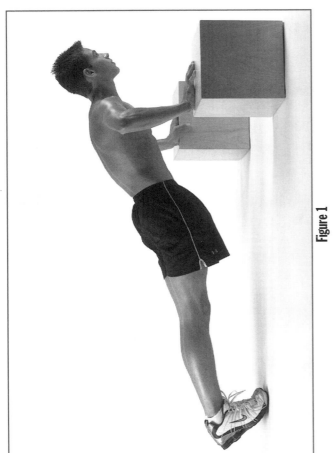

Figure 1

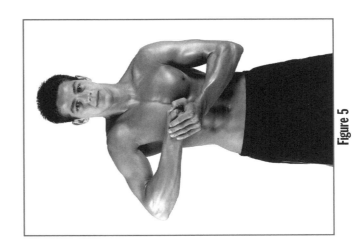

Figure 5

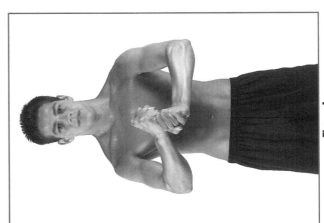

Figure 4

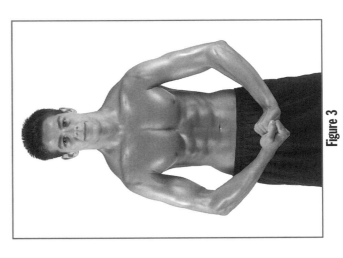

Figure 3

POWERFLEX
ABDOMINALS

FLEXERCISE
THE·TOTAL·BODY·WORKOUT

ABDOMINALS WORKOUT

You can have strong, rippling washboard abs! No equipment, weights, pulleys, or machines! Just five simple Flexercises for 20 minutes a day.

Flexercise™ for Strong, Rippling Washboard Abs

A massively muscular chest combined with deeply rippled abdominal muscles is an impressive sight. The person possessing both will always attract interest. And envy!

With consistency, determination, and patience, it's possible to build strong, well-defined abdominal muscles more quickly than you'd believe. Strengthening your abdominal muscles will help you breathe more deeply, too, which will improve your general health.

No earthly creatures that I know of have stronger, more impressive abdominal muscles than the dolphin and the shark. Imagine the incredible strength it takes for a trick-show dolphin to pull itself out of the water and "walk" across it by balancing on its tail and flexing its abdominal muscles! Talk about functional strength! Sharks, on the other hand, don't do cute tricks for tourists. Their power, speed, and ferocity have inspired respect and terror for thousands of years.

Now let's Flexercise™!

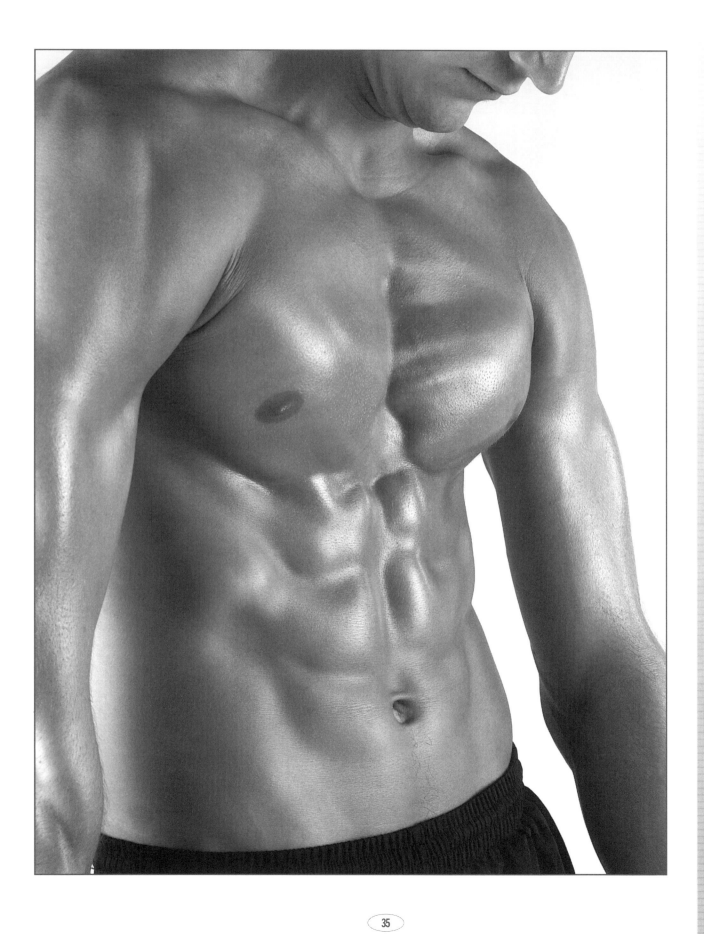

#1 DOLPHIN FLEX I

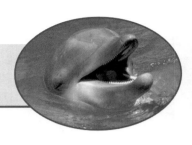

Dolphins swim by using their abdominal muscles to move their tail fins up and down. This Flexercise™ imitates that movement.

Lie flat on the floor on your back (or on an exercise mat or carpet). Put your hands under your buttocks with your palms down. Your legs should be together and straight. Keeping your legs together and straight, lift them until they're pointing straight up. Then lower them to the floor again.

LEVEL THREE: 60 repetitions
LEVEL TWO: 30 repetitions
LEVEL ONE: 15 repetitions

REMEMBER: do only as many repetitions as you can do comfortably.

ABDOMINALS

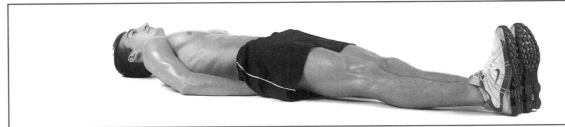

Figure 1

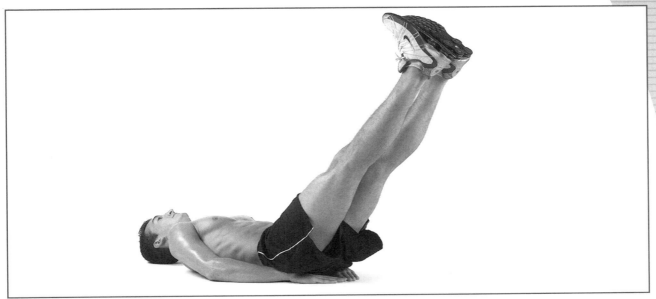

Figure 2

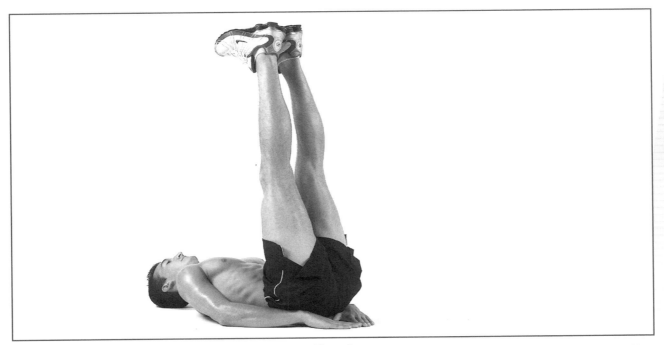

Figure 3

#2 DOLPHIN FLEX II

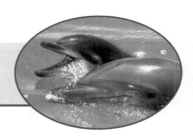

Lie flat on the floor on your back (or on an exercise mat or carpet). Keep your legs together and straight, resting the palms of your hands beside your ears. Tense your abdominal muscles and sit up as far as you can while keeping your legs on the floor. Try to touch your elbows to your knees. If you can, great. If you can't, that's okay—raise your body as far as you can without straining. This stimulates the stomach muscles, similar to the dolphin's movements.

> **LEVEL THREE:** 100 repetitions
> **LEVEL TWO:** 50 repetitions
> **LEVEL ONE:** 25 repetitions

This Flexercise™ is tough for most people—but then again, "most people" won't do the work necessary to build washboard abs. Patience and consistency are your keys. Exercise is like a bank account: you only get out of it what you put into it. And when you put a lot into it, expect to earn lots of interest!

ABDOMINALS

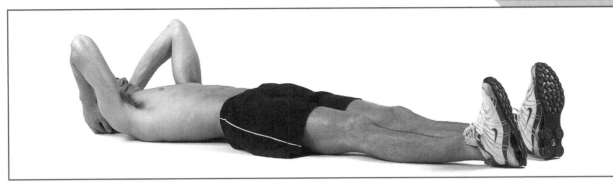

Figure 1

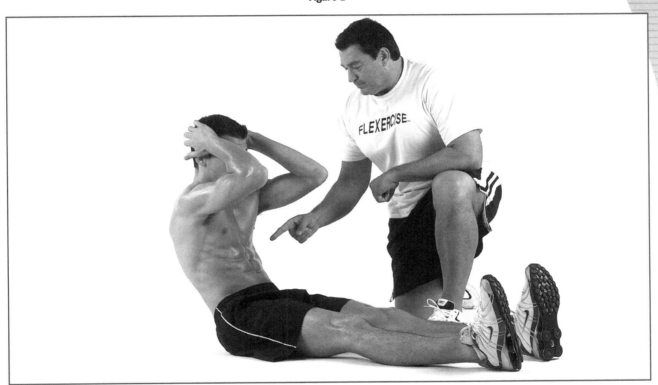

Figure 2

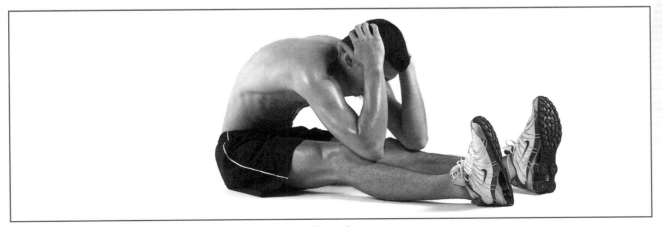

Figure 3

#3 SHARK FLEX I

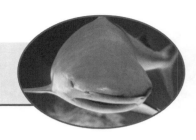

Sharks don't act like dolphins, and they don't swim like them, either. While dolphins swim by moving their tails up and down, sharks swim by moving theirs from side to side. You need to do both up-and-down and side-to-side movements to strengthen your abdominal muscles from all angles—and to deepen all the ridges in your washboard!

Lie flat on the floor on your back (or on an exercise mat or carpet). Put your hands under your buttocks with your palms down. Lift your legs until they point straight up. Now, move your feet like the shark moves its fins. Open your legs until they form a wide V, then bring them back together and cross them. Your right foot will stretch toward the left and your left foot will stretch toward the right. It's a four-part movement: up, out, cross, and down. With each repetition, alternate which leg you cross in front.

> **LEVEL THREE:** 40 repetitions
> **LEVEL TWO:** 20 repetitions
> **LEVEL ONE:** 10 repetitions

As with all Flexercises, go ahead and do your repetitions in sets, if it's easier for you that way.

ABDOMINALS

40

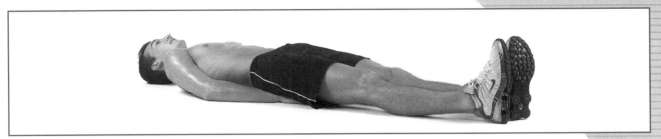

Figure 1

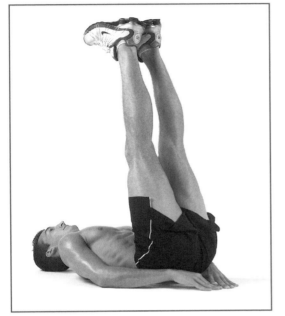

Figure 2

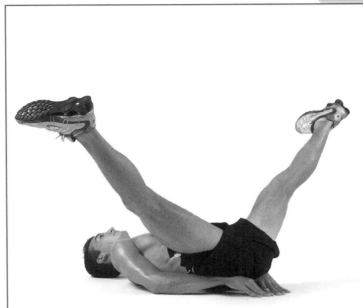

Figure 3

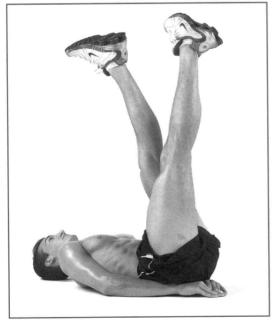

Figure 4

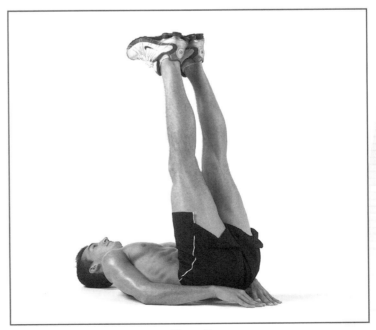

Figure 5

#4 SHARK FLEX II

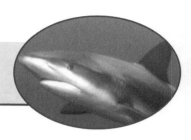

We've all seen men and women walking around with "love handles"—bulges of unsightly fat hanging above their belts at their sides. This Flexercise™ targets the obliques, the muscles underneath those "love handles." You are going to simulate the shark's side-to-side movement with your upper body.

Stand with your hands on your hips, your feet shoulder-width apart, and your legs straight. Bend to your right as far as you can without straining. Let your right hand slide down your right leg as you bend. As your right hand slides down, curl your left arm upward until it's over your head and pointing to the right. Doing this will help you bend a little farther to the right. Return to the starting position and repeat, bending to your left this time.

LEVEL THREE: 50 repetitions (25 per side)
LEVEL TWO: 30 repetitions
LEVEL ONE: 20 repetitions

Again, don't stretch farther than is comfortable for you. This Flexercise™ is very similar to one that kung fu masters have used for thousands of years to help them relax.

REMEMBER: Flexercises should feel good to do!

ABDOMINALS

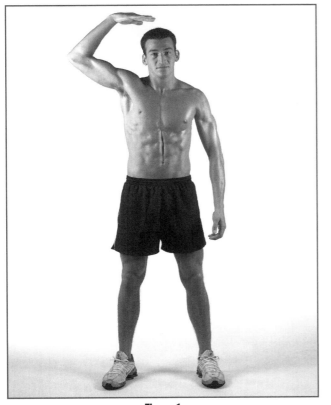

Figure 1

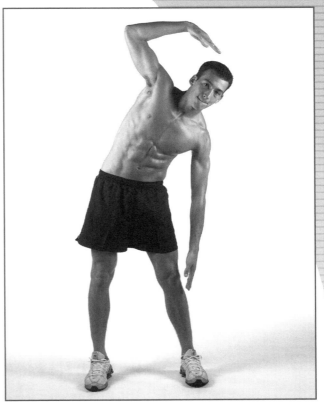

Figure 2

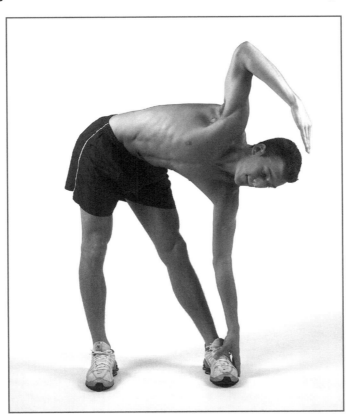

Figure 3

#5 DOLPHIN FLEX III

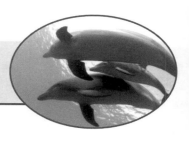

Here's one last up-and-down movement to finish your workout. First, set a sturdy chair or stool a few feet away from a heavy piece of furniture (such as a bed, dresser, or couch). Sit sideways on the chair or stool and slide your feet under the bed, dresser, or couch.

Now that you're in position, rest the palms of your hands beside your ears and lean back slowly. If you can, lean back until your body's parallel to the floor. Then tense your abdominal muscles as you sit back up.

Don't lean back farther than is comfortable for you and never bend past a 90° angle—to do so could hurt your lower back.

> **LEVEL THREE:** 100 repetitions
> **LEVEL TWO:** 50 repetitions
> **LEVEL ONE:** 25 repetitions

That's it, my friend. By practicing these five Flexercises regularly and eating sensibly, you'll build lean washboard abs where your belly used to be! Just to be clear, "eating sensibly" means eating lots of fresh vegetables and fruits, along with whole grains and lean meat. Be sure to drink plenty of water, too.

Don't be in a hurry to increase the number of repetitions you do: *doing more reps doesn't mean you're burning more fat!* There are more effective (and more enjoyable) ways to burn fat than by doing extremely high repetitions of your Flexercises. If fat burning is one of your goals, I've got you covered—just wait till you get to the Speed, Energy, and Endurance Workout later in this course!

REMEMBER: the key to success with Flexercises isn't the number of repetitions you do, but the amount of tension you use while doing them!

ABDOMINALS

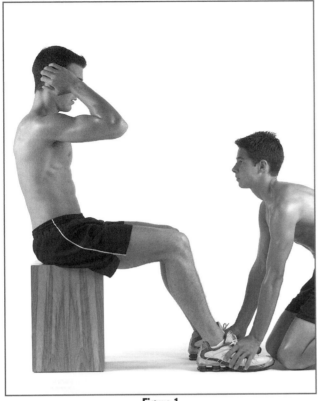

Figure 1

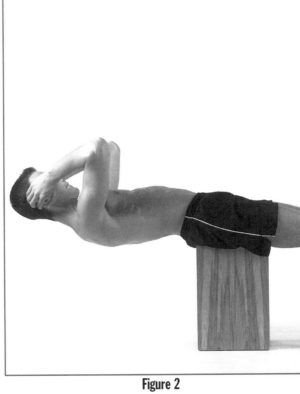

Figure 2

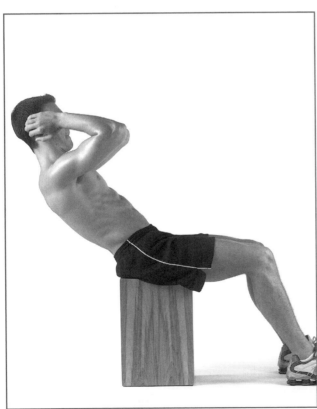

Figure 3

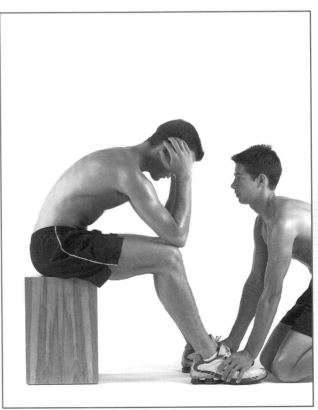

Figure 4

POWeRFLEX

ABDOMINAL EXERCISES

DOLPHIN FLEX I figure 1

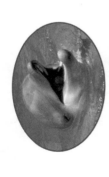

DOLPHIN FLEX II figure 2

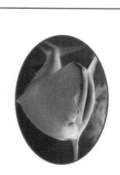

SHARK FLEX I figure 3

SHARK FLEX II figure 4

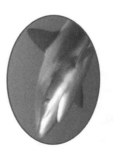

DOLPHIN FLEX III figure 5

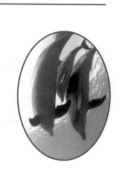

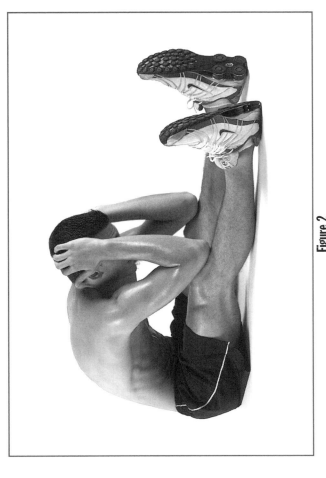

Figure 2

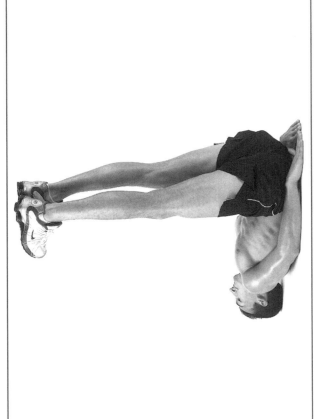

Figure 1

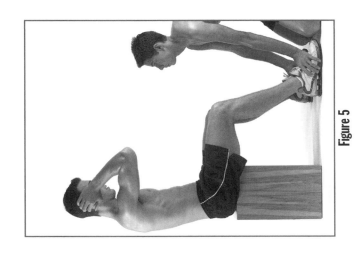

Figure 5

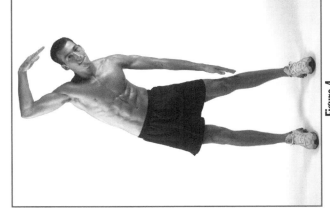

Figure 4

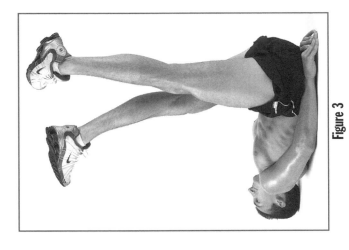

Figure 3

POWERFLEX
SPINE

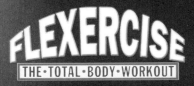

SPINE WORKOUT

You can have a healthy, flexible, energetic spine without the use of special equipment, pulleys, or machines. Just do these five Flexercises for 20 minutes a day.

Flexercise™ for a Healthy, Flexible, Energetic Spine

Like a transformer tower that holds up ultra-high power electrical lines, the human spine holds up the spinal cord, which moves electrical energy—the vitality, radiance, and power of health—through the body.

The spinal column is made up of 24 separate bones (or vertebrae) and two fused bones, the sacrum (with five bones) and the coccyx (with four bones). If any of these separate or fused bones is out of place, energy won't move through the body the way it's meant to. If energy becomes blocked, pain and illness often follow.

Any chiropractor will tell you that your health—physical and mental—depends on the health and flexibility of your spine. Yet very few other exercise courses include movements designed to protect and improve the spine's health and flexibility. The five Flexercises in this Workout imitate the movements of the eel and the alligator, two creatures whose incredibly flexible spines allow them to twist, turn, swim, and strike with purpose and power.

IMPORTANT: Do the Flexercises in this workout slowly and smoothly. Don't bend or twist any farther than is comfortable for you and don't use high tension in your muscles when doing them. These Flexercises aren't as difficult as other ones you've done, but doing them will make all the other Flexercises more effective.

Now, let's Flexercise™!

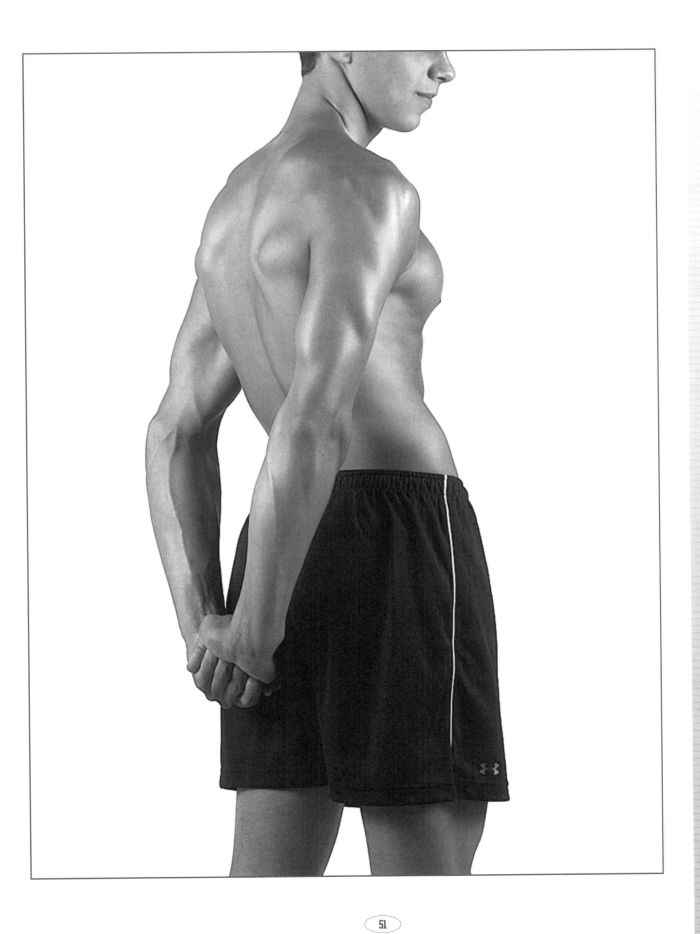

#1 EEL FLEX I

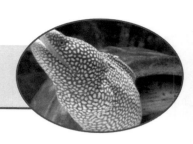

Sit on a chair or stool and fold your arms in front of you. Twist to the left from your waist as far as you can comfortably. Then return to your starting position and twist to your right. Move smoothly and take your time. Twisting to the left once and to the right once counts as one repetition.

LEVEL THREE: 40 repetitions (20 per side)
LEVEL TWO: 20 repetitions
LEVEL ONE: 10 repetitions

SPINE

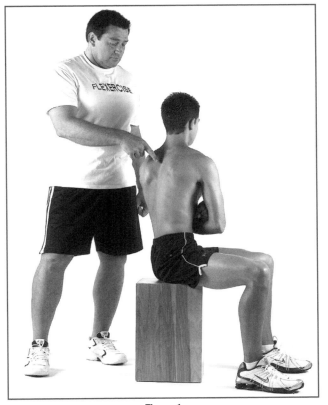

Figure 1

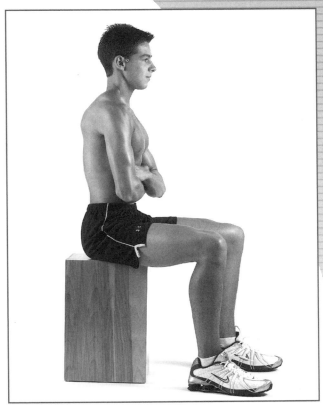

Figure 2

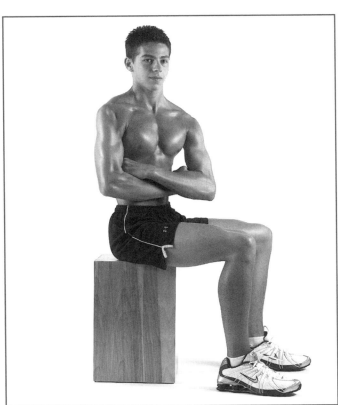

Figure 3

#2 EEL FLEX II

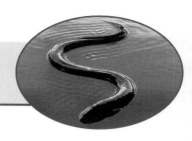

This Flexercise™ is for the upper part of the spine. While these exercises may not seem as strenuous as others, they are critical in keeping a flexible spine.

Sit or stand facing forward and bend your head down as far as you can comfortably. Try to touch your chin to the bottom of your neck. Now, move your head back as far as you can comfortably. Try to touch the back of your head to the back of your neck. Again, move smoothly. Bending forward once and back once counts as one repetition.

LEVEL THREE: 20 repetitions
LEVEL TWO: 10 repetitions
LEVEL ONE: 5 repetitions

SPINE

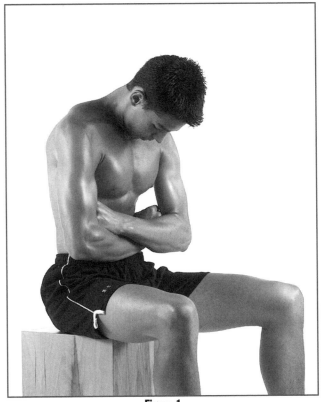

Figure 1

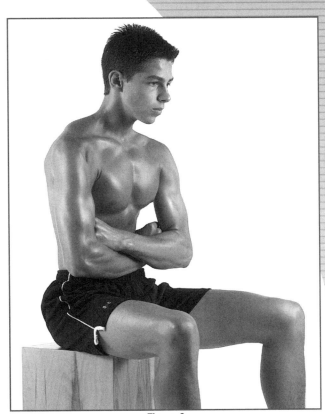

Figure 2

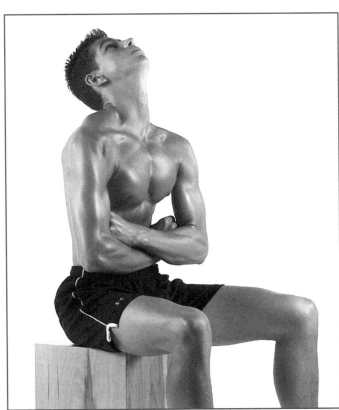

Figure 3

#3 ALLIGATOR FLEX I

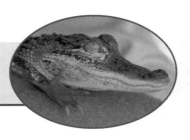

The alligator is one of Mother Nature's greatest wrestlers, and its best move is the Alligator Roll. Thanks to its flexible spine, it can pull victims toward it by rolling its body. If you don't want to become a victim of back pain, be sure to do this Flexercise™!

Stand with your feet shoulder-width apart. Clasp your hands behind your back and twist to your right as far as you can comfortably. Then repeat the movement while twisting to your left. Twisting to your right once and to your left once counts as one repetition.

> **LEVEL THREE:** 50 repetitions
> **LEVEL TWO:** 25 repetitions
> **LEVEL ONE:** 15 repetitions

SPINE

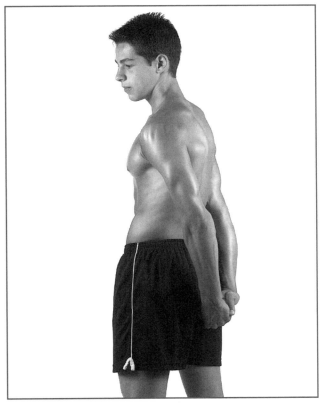

Figure 1

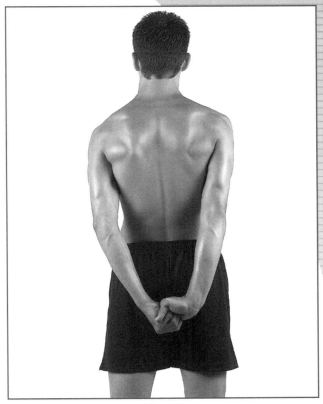

Figure 2

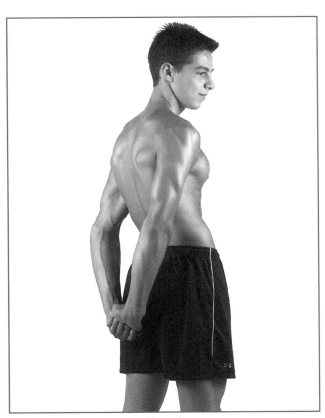

Figure 3

#4 ALLIGATOR FLEX II

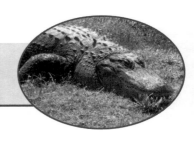

This Flexercise™ stretches your spine in two ways, with a forward bend and a backward bend. This combination stimulates the movement of energy—and health—through the spine and throughout the body.

Stand with your feet together and your knees straight. Lift your arms overhead, then bend forward as far as you can comfortably while keeping your knees straight. Stand up again smoothly, raising your hands overhead again and bending backward. Don't try to bend backward farther than is comfortable for you.

> **LEVEL THREE:** 40 repetitions
> **LEVEL TWO:** 20 repetitions
> **LEVEL ONE:** 10 repetitions

SPINE

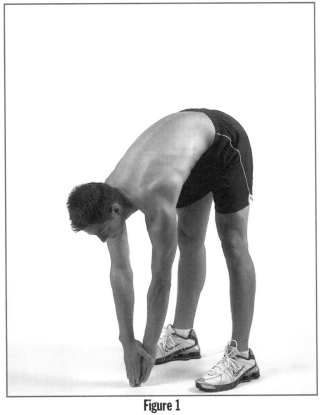

Figure 1

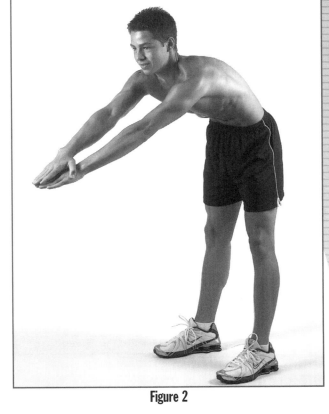

Figure 2

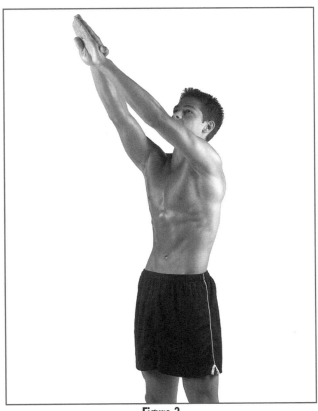

Figure 3

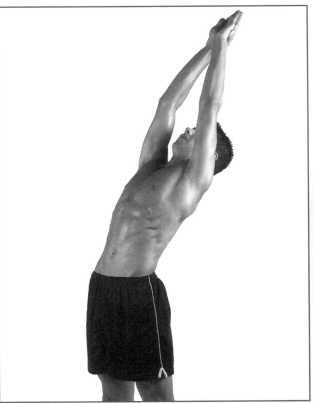

Figure 4

#5 EEL FLEX III

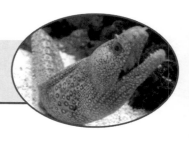

The last Flexercise™ in this workout is one more side-to-side twist. If you've noticed, the eel has no hands, arms, feet, or legs. It keeps fit and full of energy by twisting, turning, flexing, swimming, and striking—all with its body trunk. I am working your spine the same way.

Stand with your feet together, your knees straight, and your arms straight overhead. Twist from the waist as far as you can to your left, then twist as far as you can to the right.

LEVEL THREE: 40 repetitions
LEVEL TWO: 20 repetitions
LEVEL ONE: 10 repetitions

There you are, friend. Practicing these Flexercises consistently and patiently will go a long way toward protecting and improving your spine's health. Always remember that your mental and physical health depend on the health and flexibility of your spine. After all, if you want to show "backbone," you'd better have a healthy one! Now get busy!

SPINE

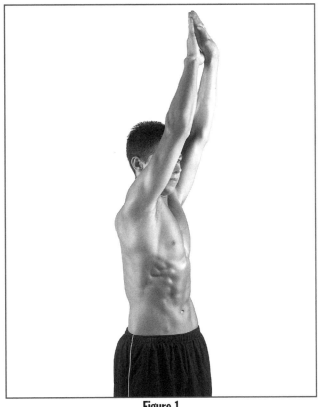

Figure 1

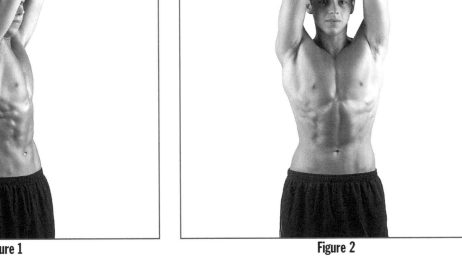

Figure 2

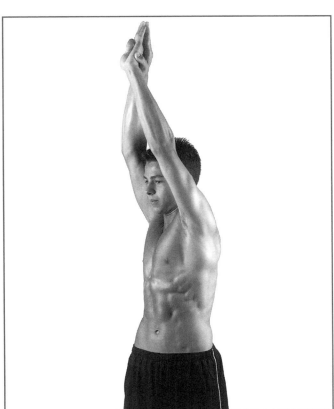

Figure 3

SPINE EXERCISES

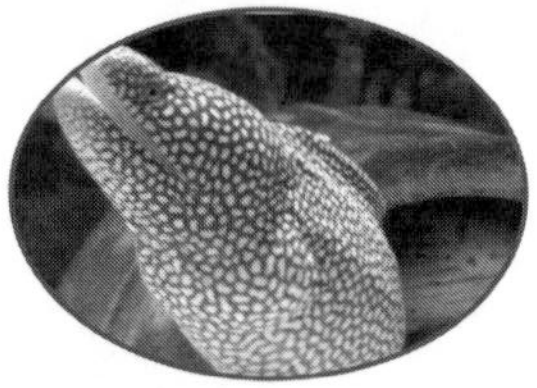

EEL FLEX I
figure 1

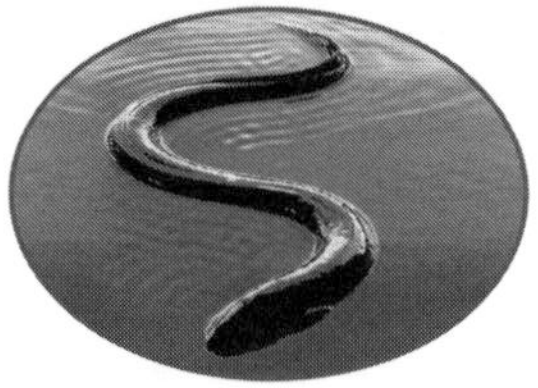

EEL FLEX II
figure 2

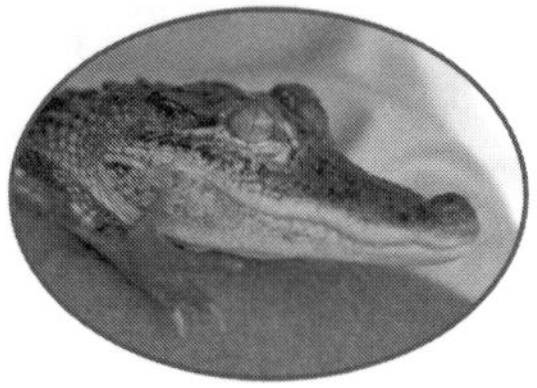

ALLIGATOR FLEX I
figure 3

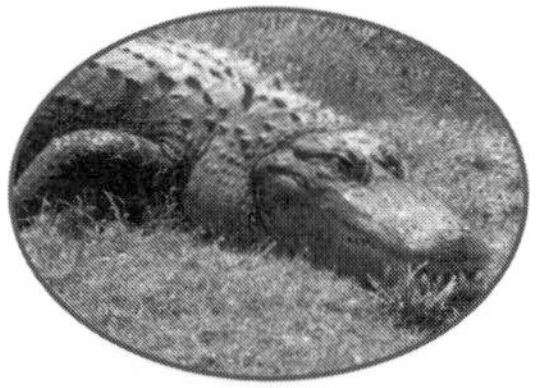

ALLIGATOR FLEX II
figure 4

EEL FLEX III
figure 5

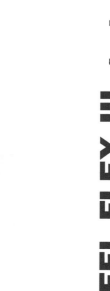
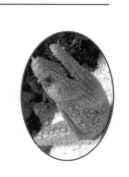

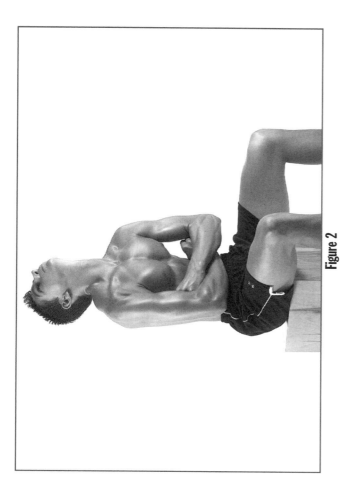

Figure 2

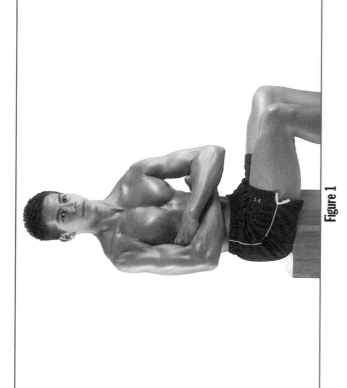

Figure 1

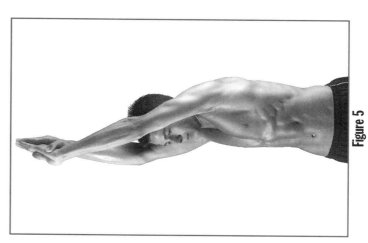

Figure 5

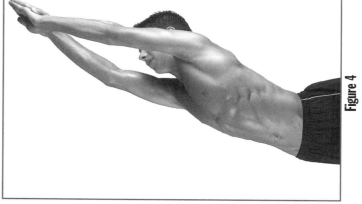

Figure 4

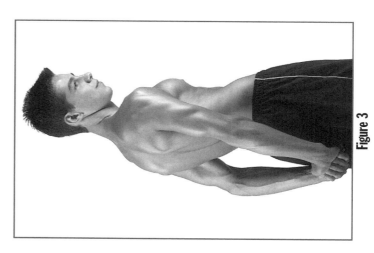

Figure 3

POWER*FLEX*
NECK

FLEXERCISE
THE·TOTAL·BODY·WORKOUT

NECK WORKOUT

You can have a firm, strong, powerful neck without using equipment, weights, pulleys, or machines. Just do five Flexercises for 20 minutes a day.

Flexercise™ for a Firm, Strong, Powerful Neck

You've probably heard tragic stories about athletes whose careers—or even lives—were ended by catastrophic neck injuries. Still, you don't have to be an athlete to suffer a neck injury. Just ask a car accident victim with whiplash.

Not all neck injuries are preventable. But whether you're a football player or martial artist, or whether you just share the road with tailgating drivers, the Flexercises in this workout can help you build a strong, muscular neck that's both injury-resistant and attractive.

These Flexercises imitate the movements of the bull and the giraffe, two animals whose necks are perfectly adapted to their needs. Thanks to its massively thick, powerful neck, the bull can use its horns to gore, ram, or toss anything in its path—including bullfighters and 200-pound rodeo riders. The giraffe's long, muscular neck allows it to pick fruit off of tall tree branches other animals can't reach, and to look graceful and elegant doing it.

IMPORTANT: for four of the five Flexercises here, you'll use one of your hands to provide resistance. To avoid injury and sore muscles as you get started, keep the resistance light. Never force your neck, and remember to breathe as you do the movements.

Now, let's Flexercise™!

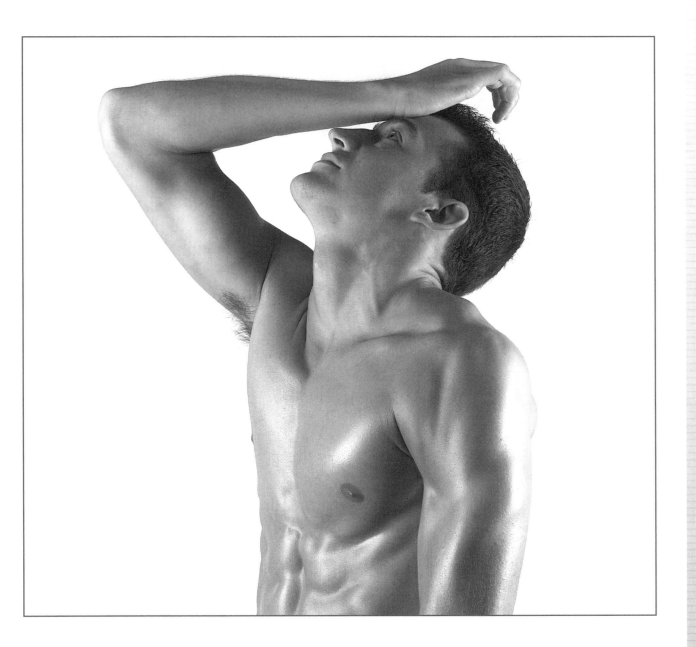

#1 BULL FLEX I

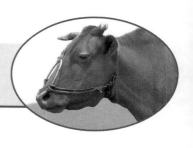

This Flexercise™ works the muscles toward the front of the neck.

Sit or stand, facing forward. Bend your head back as far as you can without straining. Place the palm of either hand on your forehead. Slowly and smoothly straighten your neck as you resist with your hand.

LEVEL THREE: 20 repetitions
LEVEL TWO: 10 repetitions
LEVEL ONE: 5 repetitions

NECK

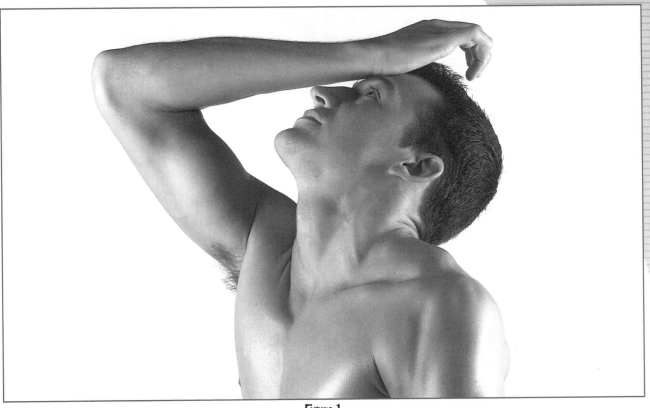

Figure 1

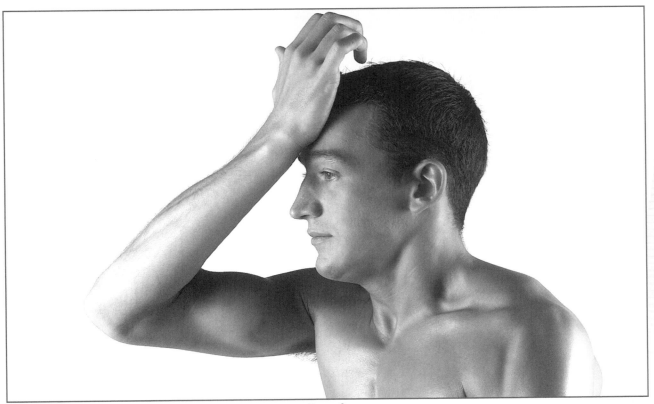

Figure 2

#2 BULL FLEX II

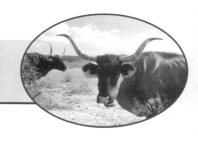

This Flexercise™ works the muscles toward the back of the neck.

Sit or stand, facing forward. Bow your head forward as far as you can without straining. Place the palm of either hand against the back of your head. Slowly and smoothly straighten your neck as you resist with your hand.

LEVEL THREE: 20 repetitions
LEVEL TWO: 10 repetitions
LEVEL ONE: 5 repetitions

NECK

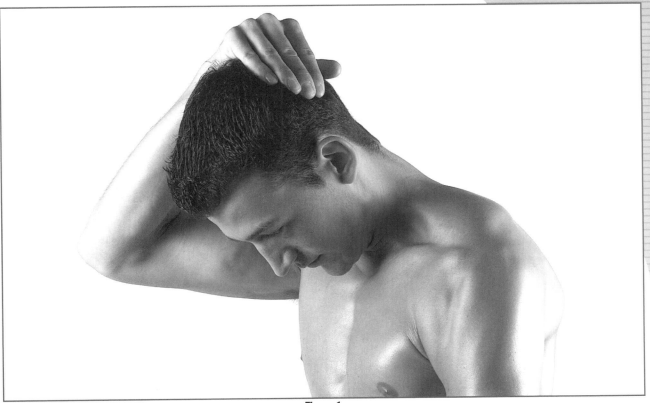

Figure 1

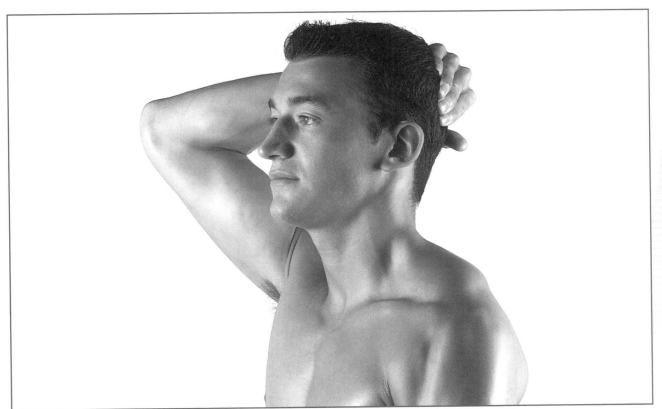

Figure 2

#3 BULL FLEX III

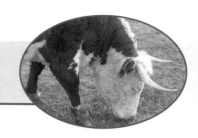

The next two Flexercises work the muscles along the sides of the neck. If you want to build a neck that's strong and attractive, it's very important to work your neck through its complete range of motion.

Sit or stand, facing forward. Bow your head down and to the right as far as you can without straining. Place the palm of your left hand on the left side of your head, just above the ear. Slowly and smoothly straighten your neck as you resist. Then reverse the movement, bowing your head down and left and resisting with your right hand as you straighten your neck again.

LEVEL THREE: 40 repetitions (20 per side)
LEVEL TWO: 20 repetitions
LEVEL ONE: 10 repetitions

NECK

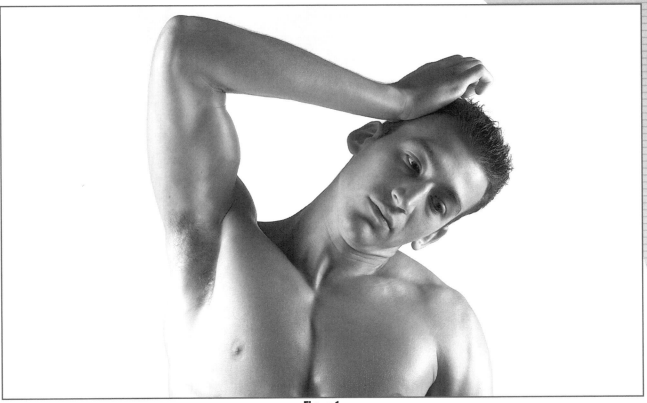

Figure 1

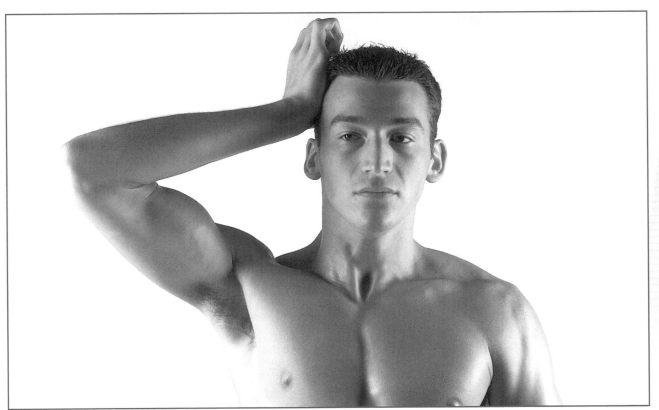

Figure 2

#4 GIRAFFE FLEX I

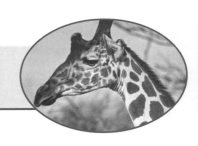

Sit or stand, facing forward. Keeping your neck straight, turn your head to the left. Place your right palm on the right side of your forehead. Slowly and smoothly turn your head, resisting with your right hand, until you're facing forward again. Switch hands and reverse the movement.

LEVEL THREE: 40 repetitions (20 per side)
LEVEL TWO: 20 repetitions
LEVEL ONE: 10 repetitions

NECK

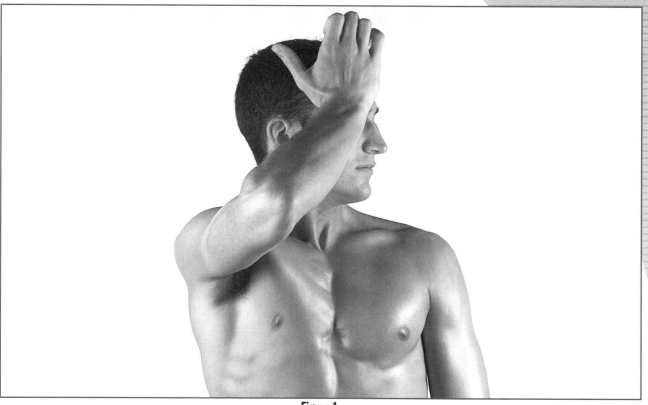

Figure 1

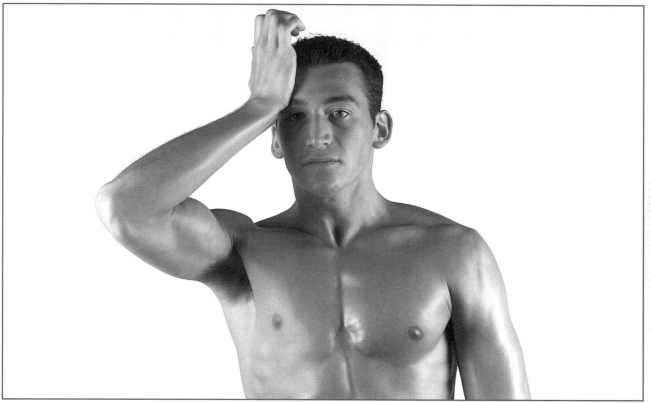

Figure 2

#5 GIRAFFE FLEX II

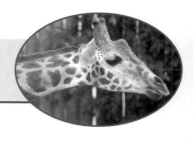

This Flexercise™ will give your neck a good stretch as you complete the workout.

Sit or stand, facing forward. Bow your head to the right as far as you can without straining. Slowly roll your head, rotating your neck in clockwise circles. Reverse the movement and repeat, rotating your neck counter-clockwise.

> **LEVEL THREE:** 20 repetitions (10 each way)
> **LEVEL TWO:** 15 repetitions
> **LEVEL ONE:** 10 repetitions

There you go: five Flexercises to help you build a strong, well-muscled, attractive neck. These Flexercises aren't hard to do. But if you do them consistently and patiently, you'll help protect your neck from injury. Build a neck worthy of a bull or a giraffe—not a chicken!

NECK

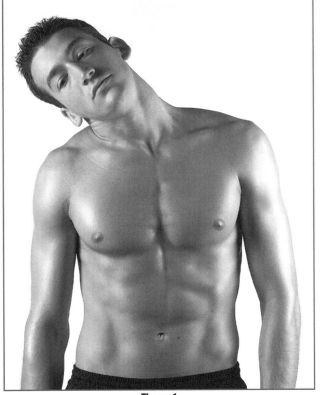
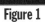

Figure 1

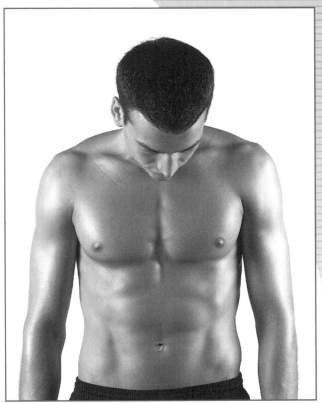

Figure 2

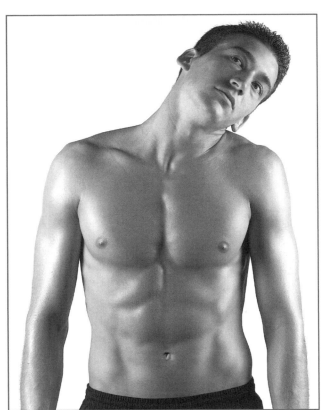

Figure 3

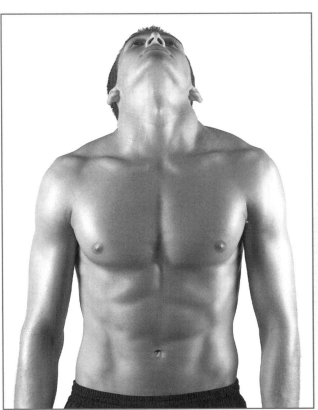

Figure 4

NECK EXERCISES

BULL FLEX I
figure 1

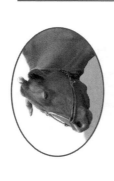

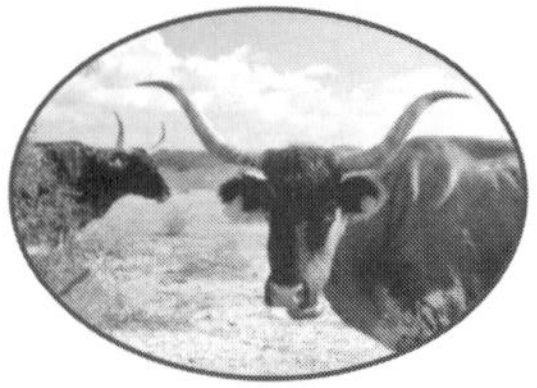

BULL FLEX II
figure 2

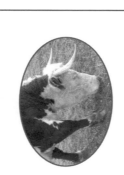

BULL FLEX II
figure 3

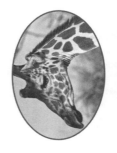

GIRAFFE FLEX I
figure 4

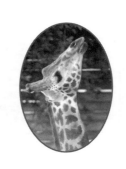

GIRAFFE FLEX II
figure 5

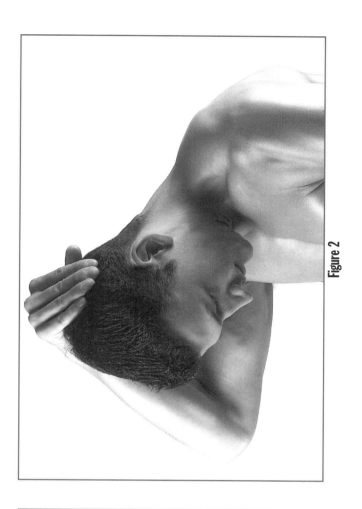

Figure 2

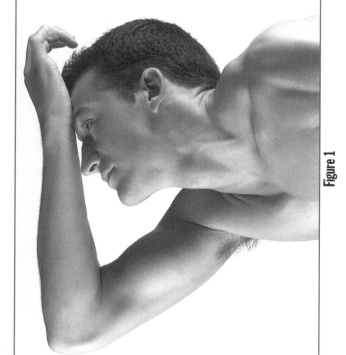

Figure 5

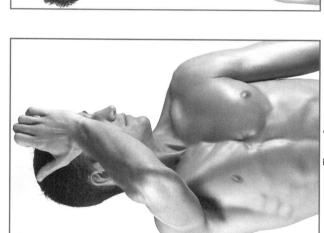

Figure 4

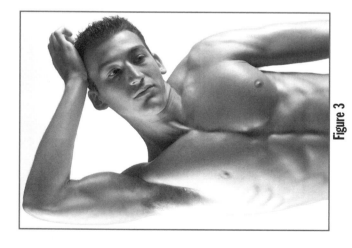

Figure 3

Figure 1

79

*POWER*FLEX
BACK

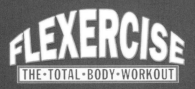

BACK WORKOUT

You can have a muscular, attractive, powerful back without using equipment, weights, pulleys, or machines. Just do five Flexercises for 20 minutes a day.

Flexercise™ for a Muscular, V-Shaped Back

For thousands of years, one of the hallmarks of a fit, healthy man or woman has been a V-shaped upper body—the striking effect created by well-developed chest and back muscles tapering down to lean, rippled abs. This look fascinated ancient Greek and Roman sculptors, who celebrated it in statues chiseled to adorn the halls of palaces. And it fascinates fashion designers today, prompting them to pay V-shaped men and women thousands of dollars a day to model their clothes for magazines and catalogs.

In the animal kingdom, no creature has been more celebrated by artists than the horse for its awe-inspiring combination of speed, power, endurance, and graceful muscularity. Civilization itself has been built on the horse's broad, sinewy back as it has carried riders and pulled carriages, chariots, wagons, and plows. Few people own horses these days, but the engines in our cars and trucks are still rated according to their horsepower.

The Flexercises in this workout imitate the movements of the horse and its diesel-powered cousin, the mule. Practicing these Flexercises with consistency, determination, and patience will give your back new strength to bear your burdens, whatever they are—and without burdening you with the crippling injuries that barbells, dumb-bells, and weight machines can cause.

Ready? Let's Flexercise™!

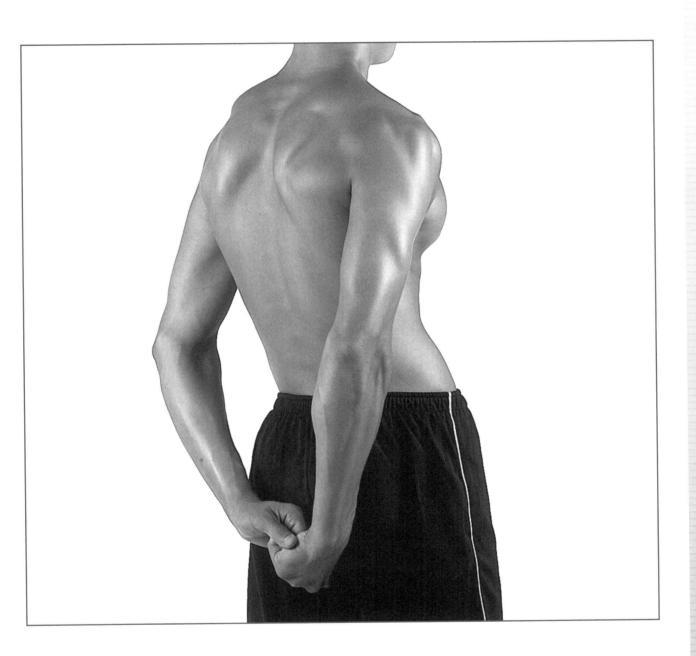

POWERFLEX

#1 HORSE FLEX I

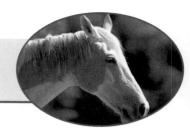

This Flexercise™ simulates the way horses' back muscles work as they pull heavy loads. It will help you improve your balance, too.

Stand with your feet shoulder-width apart. Lean over and interlock your fingers behind your left knee, just above where it bends. Stand up slowly and smoothly, resisting with your left leg as you lift it. Do an equal number of repetitions as you resist with your right leg.

LEVEL THREE: 40 repetitions (20 each side)
LEVEL TWO: 20 repetitions
LEVEL ONE: 10 repetitions

BACK

84

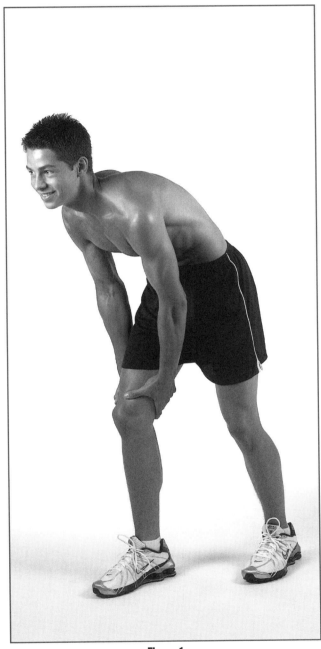

Figure 1

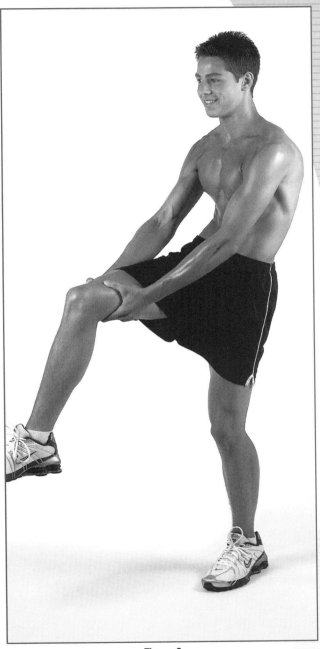

Figure 2

#2 HORSE FLEX II

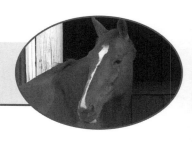

To many fans, bucking bronco horses are the stars of the rodeo. "Broncs" explode out of the chute, their backs flexing and whipping as their riders hold on for dear life. Your next Flexercise™ imitates the bronco's movement, but you won't need a rider.

First, set a sturdy chair or stool a few feet away from a heavy piece of furniture, such as a bed, dresser, or couch (you may be able to use the same setup you used for Dolphin Flex III in the Abdominal Workout). Lay face down across the chair or stool and slide your feet under the bed, dresser, or couch. Place both hands behind your head, one atop the other. Slowly and smoothly, raise your upper body as far as possible. Then lower yourself.

> **LEVEL THREE:** 50 repetitions
> **LEVEL TWO:** 25 repetitions
> **LEVEL ONE:** 10 repetitions

It's okay if you can't raise your upper body very far at first. Do the best you can. With time, your strength and range of motion will increase. Just don't give up! This Flexercise™ is essential for building a strong, healthy, pain-free lower back.

BACK

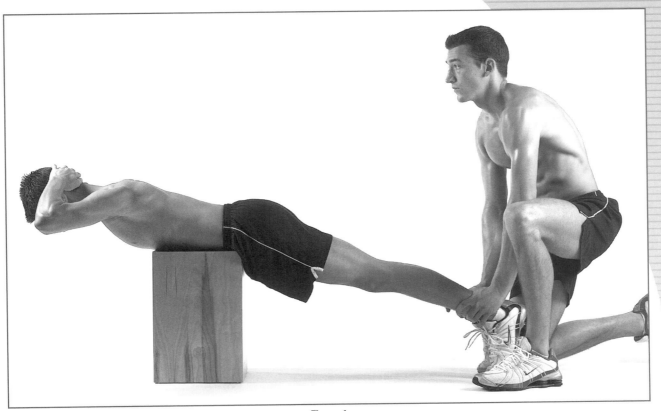

Figure 1

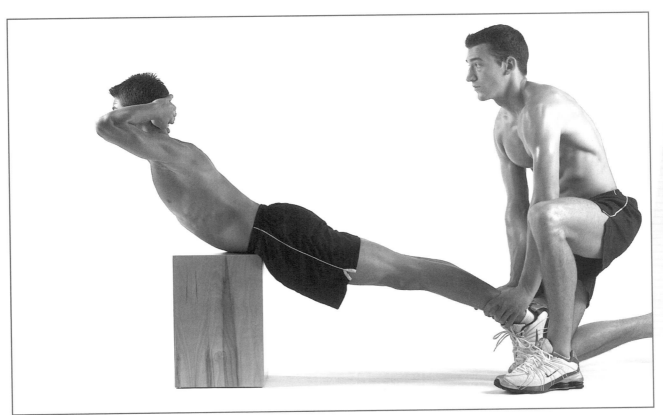

Figure 2

#3 HORSE FLEX III

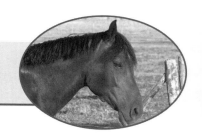

Horses are undeniably graceful, from the way they run at the Kentucky Derby to the way they brush flies off their backs by flexing the muscles at the base of their necks. This Flexercise™ imitates that movement (without the flies, of course) and works the upper back muscles.

Stand with your feet shoulder-width apart. Clasp your hands together behind your back at about waist height. Now push your shoulders back and down. Return to the starting position and repeat.

Put a little extra effort into it and your muscles will really stand out. It may seem a little awkward at first, but do them with confidence and the movements will feel very natural after a short time. You will be amazed and pleased by the results—a strong, powerful, muscular back. Envision the goal of how you want to look while you are doing your Flexercises. It will help you put a little something into your workout and help you attain your goal. Keep at it. You can have the body you want. It is attainable. Just don't quit!

LEVEL THREE: 20 repetitions
LEVEL TWO: 10 repetitions
LEVEL ONE: 5 repetitions

BACK

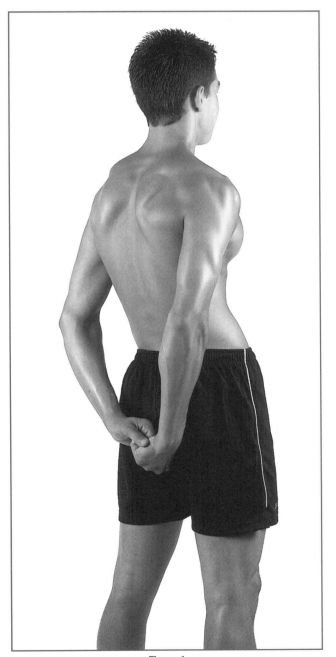

Figure 1

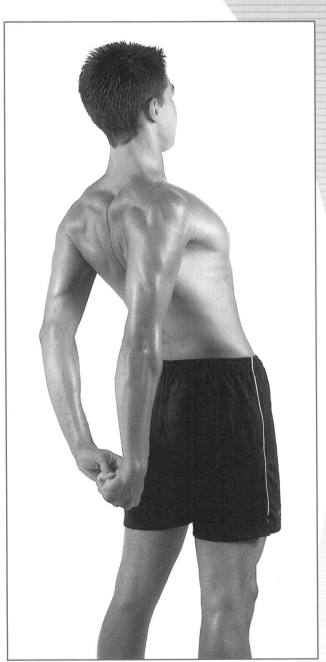

Figure 2

#4 HORSE FLEX IV

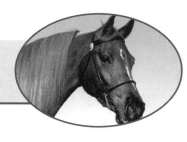

You'll look a little like a lucky horseshoe as you do this Flexercise™. Practice it faithfully, however, and you won't need luck to keep your lower back strong and healthy.

Lie face down on a soft carpet or mat. Clasp your hands behind your back. Slowly and smoothly arch your back and, at the same time, raise your legs. Pause for a moment and feel your muscles tense. Lower your torso and legs and repeat.

> **LEVEL THREE:** 15 repetitions
> **LEVEL TWO:** 10 repetitions
> **LEVEL ONE:** 5 repetitions

Similar to Horse Flex II, this one can be difficult at first. It takes practice to coordinate the movements, but keep at it. Your coordination will improve with your strength. Remember that with Flexercise™, tension is always more important than repetition—one perfect repetition is worth much more than 15 sloppy ones.

BACK

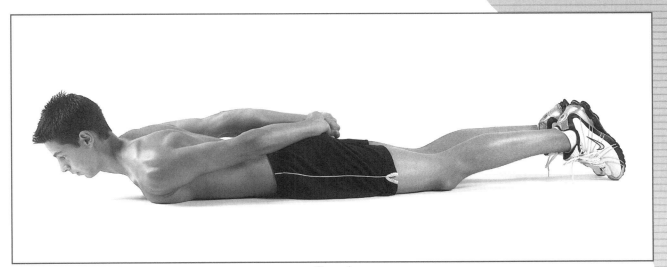

Figure 1

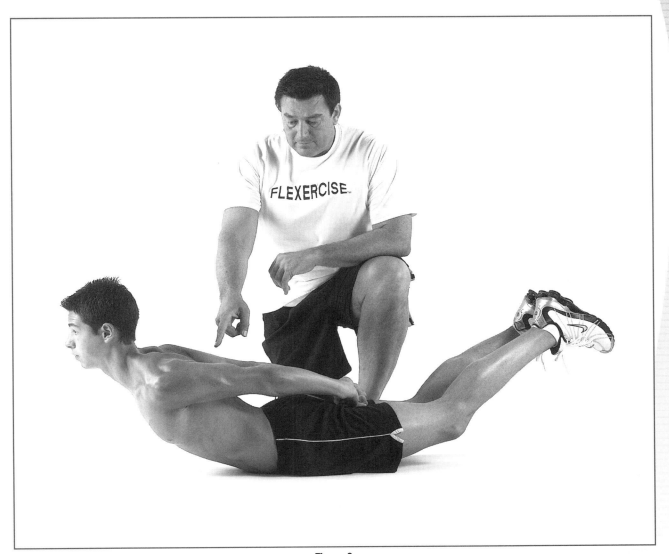

Figure 2

#5 MULE FLEX

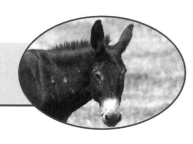

Unlike the horse, the mule isn't known for its grace but for the raw strength it uses to carry and pull immense loads that would break other creatures' backs. The last Flexercise™ in this workout imitates the way the mule bends and straightens itself beneath a load.

Stand with your feet shoulder-width apart. Keeping your legs straight, slowly and smoothly bend forward. Touch your toes, if you can do so without straining. Stand up again slowly and smoothly and raise your hands above your head, extending your arms as far as you can to either side. Bend backward slightly. Keeping your arms straight, push them toward each other. Hold this position for a moment, then lower your arms and repeat.

LEVEL THREE: 15 repetitions
LEVEL TWO: 10 repetitions
LEVEL ONE: 5 repetitions

There you go, friend. Practiced with consistency, determination, and patience, these five Flexercises will not only stretch and strengthen every muscle in your back but will teach your body to coordinate and use that strength—something pumping iron won't do. Whatever your burdens, may you stand straight, tall, and proud for as long as you live…with strength, health, and Flexercise™!

BACK

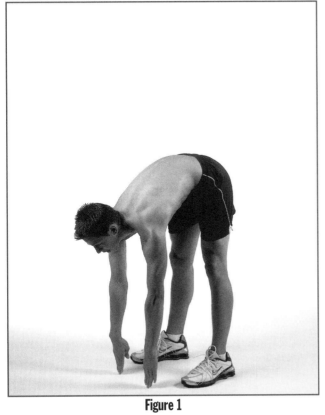

Figure 1

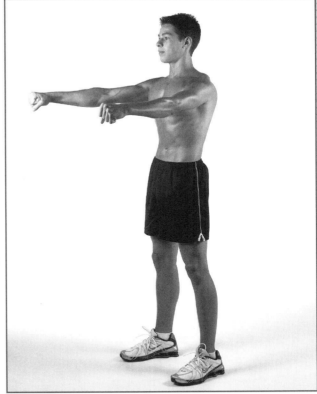

Figure 2

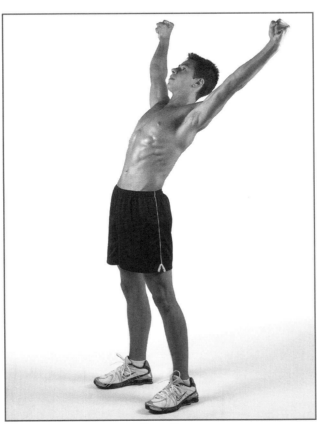

Figure 3

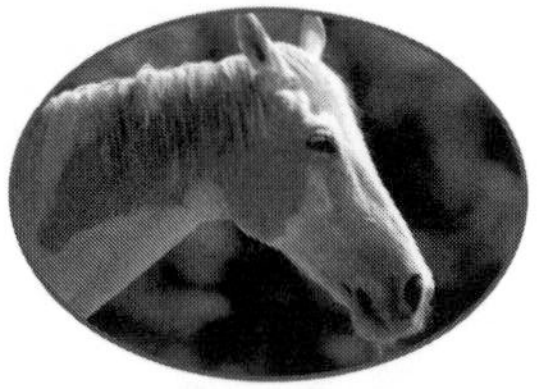

POWERFLEX

BACK EXERCISES

HORSE FLEX I
figure 1

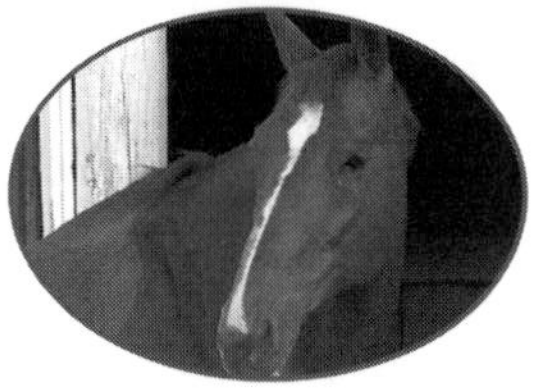

HORSE FLEX II
figure 2

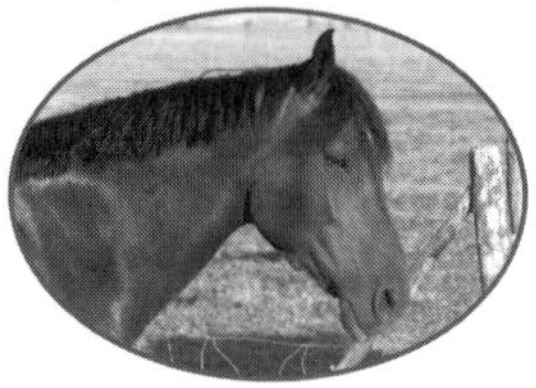

HORSE FLEX III
figure 3

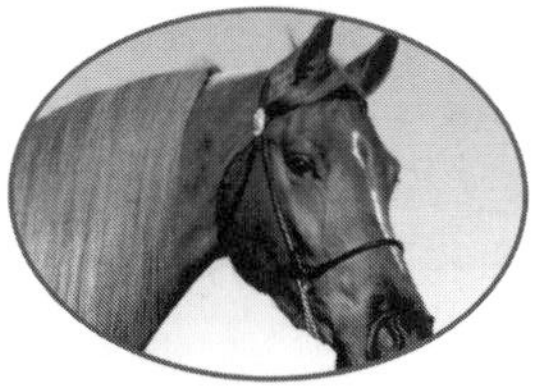

HORSE FLEX IV
figure 4

MULE FLEX
figure 5

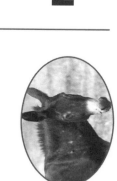

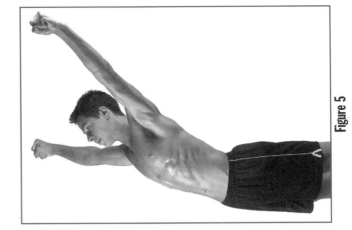

Figure 2

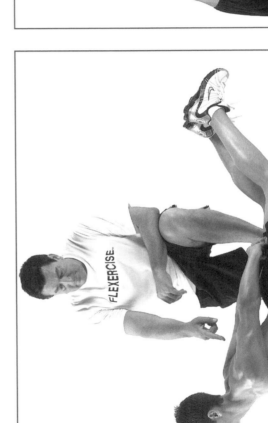

Figure 3

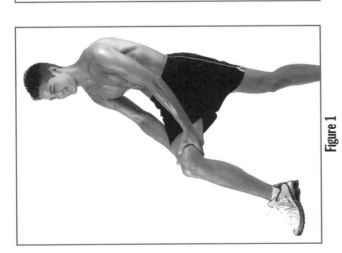

Figure 1

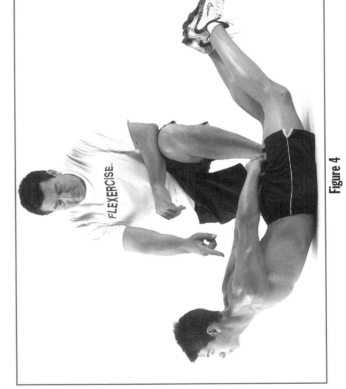

Figure 4

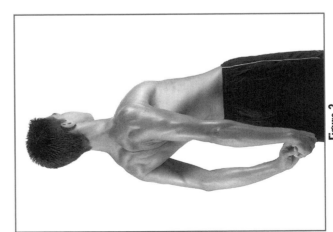

Figure 5

TAKING STOCK

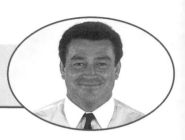

Dear Friend,

Now that you're halfway through this Flexercise™ course, it's an excellent time to take stock. Remind yourself of where you've come from, where you are, and where you're going.

If you're following the Workout rotation I recommended earlier, you've been practicing the Chest Workout for the last four weeks and have practiced the Abdominal, Spine, Neck, and Back Workouts for a week each. By now, you've begun to reap the rewards of consistent, determined, and patient Flexercise™.

What do you see? Are your eyes brighter and clearer? As you look at yourself in the mirror after taking a shower, maybe your chest, shoulders, and arms seem larger and better defined. Maybe your shirts seem too tight in the chest and arms…and too loose in the waist! Maybe when you're stuck in traffic you catch yourself flexing your abs or biceps…just because it feels good.

And how do you feel? Maybe you sleep better. Maybe it's easier to carry bags of groceries, or to weed the garden, mow the lawn, or stack firewood. Maybe you feel more graceful, more confident in your movements, as you vacuum the living room. At the end of the day, maybe you don't feel as tired.

If you've experienced results such as these, you aren't the only one who's noticed. What have your coworkers said? What have your friends and family members said? Have they asked you whether you're lifting weights? Or which gym you've joined?

Friend, I commend you for your courage. It takes courage to identify changes you want to make, and it takes even more courage to make positive, healthy changes into healthy habits, as you have. I feel blessed that, through Flexercise™, I've had this opportunity to help you begin to see and feel the body you were always meant to have.

As you continue this course, be proud of what you've accomplished. As you learn the Flexercises in the remaining Workouts, remember to keep building your "mind-muscle connection." As your muscles work, imagine them as you want them to look and feel. And be sure that with Flexercise™, your best is always yet to come!

Once more, congratulations!

Sincerely,

Jim Forystek
Creator, Flexercise™

POWERFLEX
LEGS

LEGS WORKOUT

You can have powerful, strong, attractive, muscular legs without using equipment, weights, pulleys, or machines. Just do five Flexercises for 20 minutes a day.

Flexercise™ for Tireless, Attractive, Explosively Athletic Legs

As you begin the second half of this Flexercise™ course, it's no accident that the next workout is for the your legs. After all, the legs contain some of the human body's largest, strongest muscles. In fact, having strong, healthy legs is so fundamental to our health and fitness that exercises designed to develop the legs also stimulate muscle development throughout the body. When your thighs get bigger and stronger, your chest, shoulders, and arms do, too!

Every athlete knows that leg power and endurance are often the difference between victory and defeat on the field, court, and mat. Muscular, athletic legs attract attention on the sidewalk and at the beach, too, prompting turns and whistles by members of both sexes. And when a song or movie has been popular for a while, entertainment people say it "has legs."

Horses, lions, panthers, and antelopes all run swiftly, thanks to their strong legs. But I think the most impressive legs in the animal kingdom belong to jumpers: to the frog and the kangaroo. Sure, frogs are small and green, but their explosively powerful legs allow them to jump distances many times their own length and to "frog kick" gracefully through the water when they swim. Kangaroos may look cuddly and harmless, but don't be fooled—they can jump for miles at high speed to escape their enemies, even while carrying their young in their pouches. And when the kangaroo leans back on its thick tail, one kick of its ferociously powerful legs can kill a full-grown man.

So here's to the frog and the kangaroo, two creatures whose movements we imitate in the following Flexercises.

Now, get hoppin' and Flexercise™!

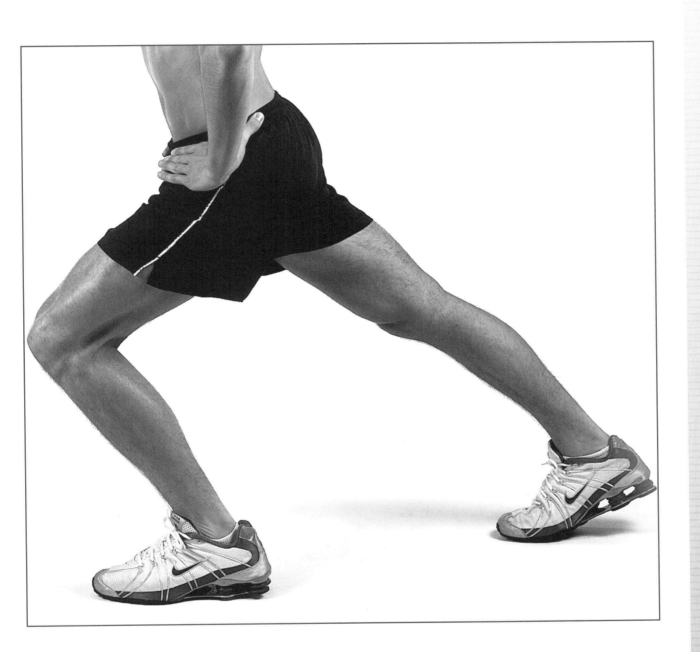

POWERFLEX

#1 FROG FLEX I

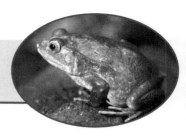

For this Flexercise™ you'll imitate the frog's position as it springs off the ground—but without becoming airborne yourself.

Stand with your heels close together and your toes pointing outward, forming a V. Place your hands on your hips and rise onto the balls of your feet. Keeping your back straight, bend your knees and lower your body as far as you can comfortably. Stay on the balls of your feet. Stand up again slowly and smoothly and repeat.

> **LEVEL THREE:** 100 repetitions
> **LEVEL TWO:** 50 repetitions
> **LEVEL ONE:** 25 repetitions

Balance can be tricky with this one. If you can't keep your hands on your hips and lower yourself without keeling over, it's okay to hold on to the back of a chair as you learn. As your confidence and strength improve, you'll find you won't need the chair. This Flexercise™ not only works your legs completely but also improves your balance.

LEGS

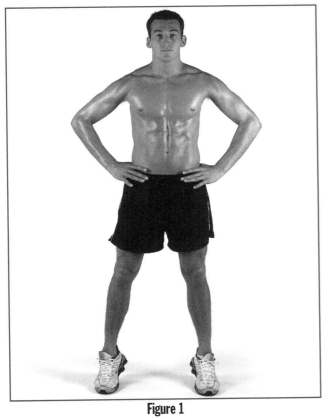

Figure 1

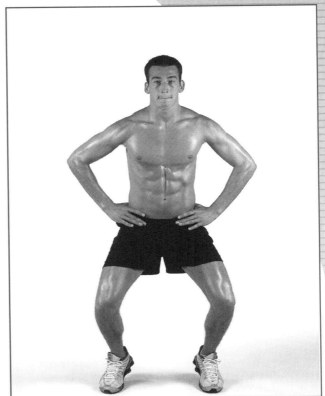

Figure 2

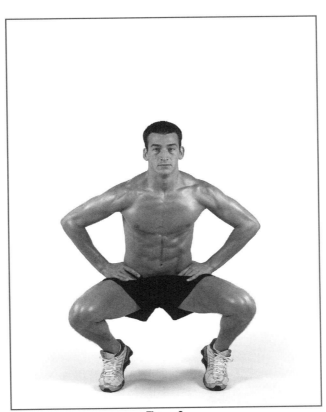

Figure 3

#2 FROG FLEX II

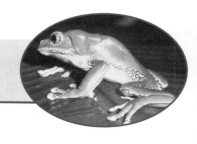

Here's a two-part Flexercise™ for the inner and outer thighs.

First, squat down as far as you can comfortably—as though you're playing leapfrog—with your knees spread wide apart. Place the palms of your hands on the inside of your knees. Now try to push your knees together while resisting with your hands. Push and resist for a second or two, then relax and repeat.

For Part Two, squat down with your knees together. Place your palms on the outside of your knees. Try to push your knees apart while resisting with your hands. Push and resist for a second or two, then relax and repeat.

> **LEVEL THREE:** 40 repetitions (20 for each part)
> **LEVEL TWO:** 20 repetitions
> **LEVEL ONE:** 10 repetitions

Be sure to apply enough tension to make this Flexercise™ challenging.

REMEMBER: Success with Flexercise™ begins with tension, not repetition! Manage the tension carefully so that every repetition is your best!

LEGS

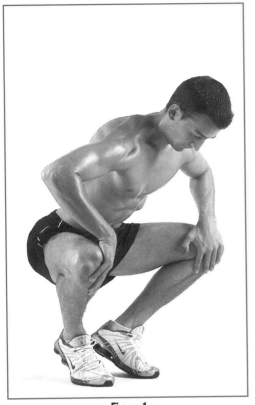

Figure 1

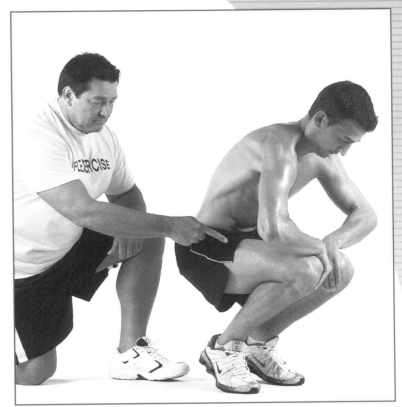

Figure 2

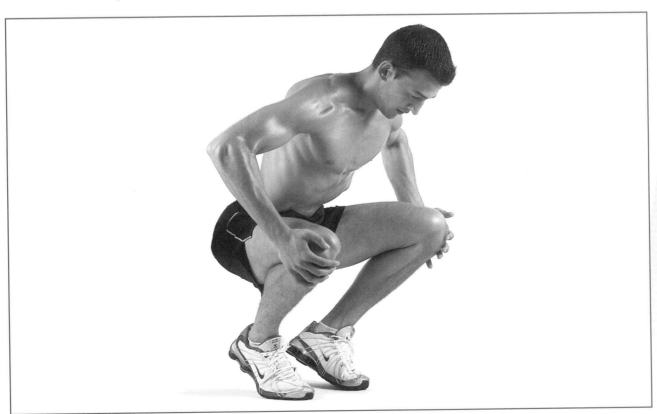

Part Two

POWERFLEX

#3 KANGAROO FLEX I

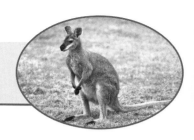

This Flexercise™ simulates the kangaroo's position as it jumps, as Frog Flex I does the frog's.

While standing, cross your legs (like a scissors), distributing your weight evenly on both feet. Hold your arms straight out in front of you. With your back straight, bend your knees and slowly lower your body as far as you can comfortably. Stand up again slowly and smoothly and repeat.

> **LEVEL THREE:** 20 repetitions
> **LEVEL TWO:** 10 repetitions
> **LEVEL ONE:** 5 repetitions

If holding your arms in front of you doesn't help you keep your balance, it's okay to hold on to the back of a chair as you learn this Flexercise™.

LEGS

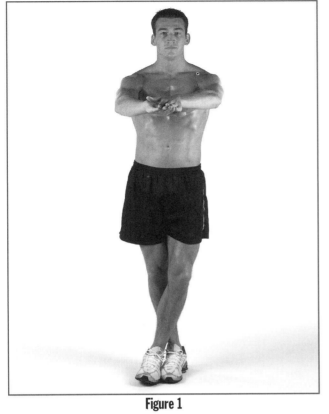

Figure 1

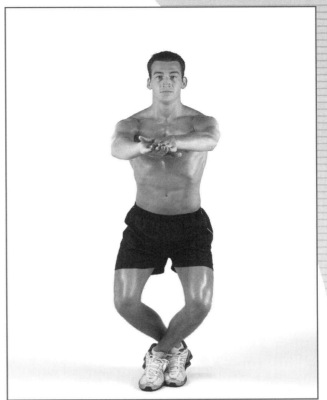

Figure 2

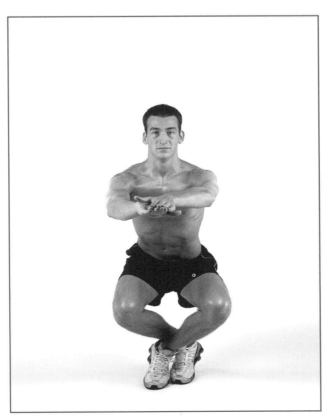

Figure 3

#4 FROG FLEX III

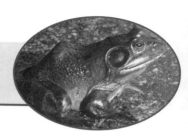

Thanks to its webbed feet and powerful legs, the frog is an excellent swimmer—so excellent that militaries around the world refer to their scuba divers as "frogmen." Your next Flexercise™ simulates the up-and-down movement of the frog's legs as it kicks through the water.

We'll work the right leg first. Stand with your feet shoulder-width apart and your hands on your hips. Without moving your left foot, step back with your right foot. Keep your right leg straight and rest the ball of your right foot on the floor. Bend your left knee slightly. Keeping your right leg straight, push down on the floor with your right foot and lean forward on to your bent left leg. Hold this position for a second or two. Straighten your left leg and repeat. Reverse the movement to work your left leg.

LEVEL THREE: 40 repetitions (20 for each leg)
LEVEL TWO: 20 repetitions
LEVEL ONE: 10 repetitions

LEGS

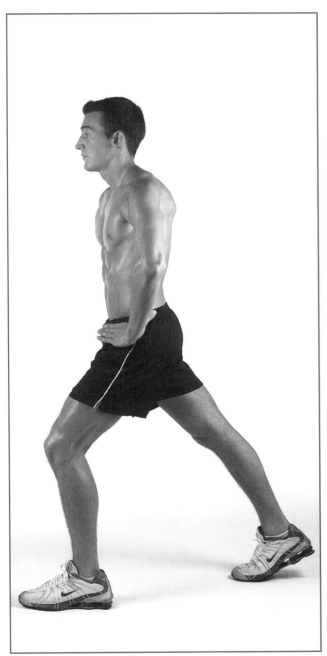

Figure 1

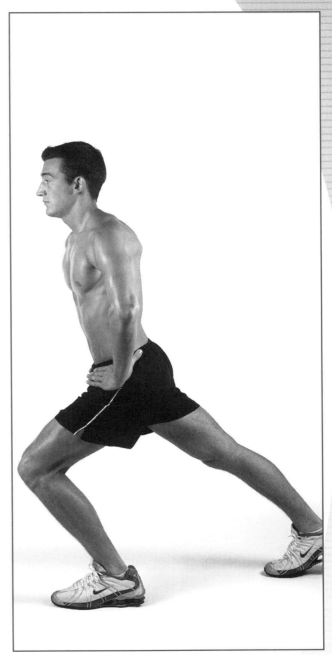

Figure 2

#5 KANGAROO FLEX II

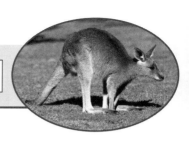

Not only does the kangaroo kick with ferocious power, but also with remarkable flexibility and control—a combination any karate master would envy. This three-part kicking Flexercise™ will help you develop these qualities.

Part One: stand with your feet shoulder-width apart. Your arms hang at your sides, or you can hang on to a chair for balance. Step backward with your right leg, then kick your right leg forward and as high as you can without straining. Keep you right leg straight as you kick. Repeat the movement, kicking with your left leg.

Part Two: same starting position as in Part One. This time, kick your right leg upward and to the left, swinging it from left to right in a circular motion.

Part Three: same starting position as in Parts One and Two. Now, kick your right leg upward and to the right, swinging it from right to left in a circular motion.

LEVEL THREE: 60 repetitions (20 per leg in each position)
LEVEL TWO: 40 repetitions
LEVEL ONE: 20 repetitions

Friend, there you have it—a complete Flexercise™ Workout to strengthen, stretch, and shape every muscle in your legs, from your toes to your thighs. With consistency, determination, and patience, you can develop legs that will carry you with confidence, whether you're wearing a football uniform, a business suit, or a bathing suit. See yourself achieving your goals, and see how Flexercise™ helps you achieve them!

LEGS

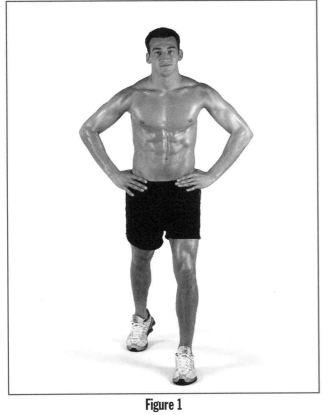

Figure 1

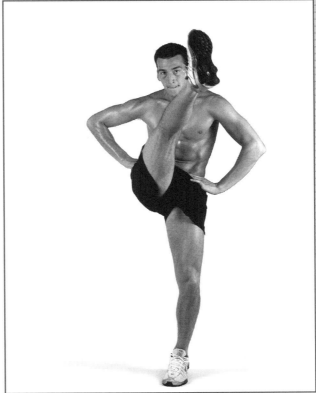

Figure 2

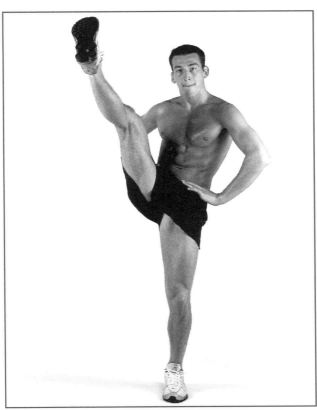

Figure 3

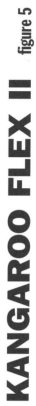

LEG EXERCISES

FROG FLEX I
figure 1

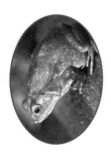

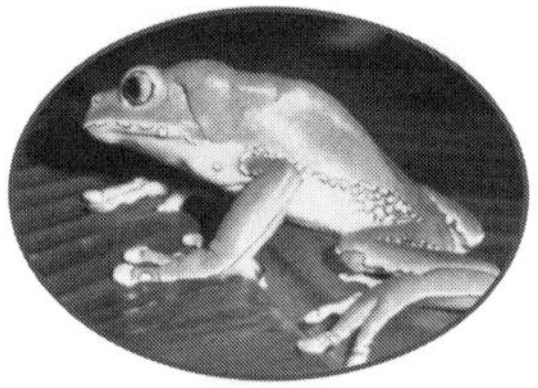

FROG FLEX II
figure 2

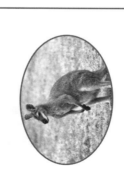

KANGAROO FLEX I
figure 3

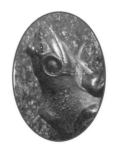

FROG FLEX III
figure 4

KANGAROO FLEX II
figure 5

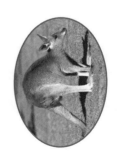

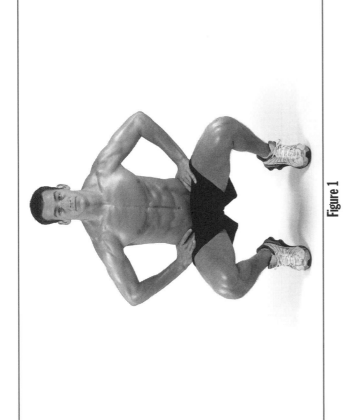

Figure 1

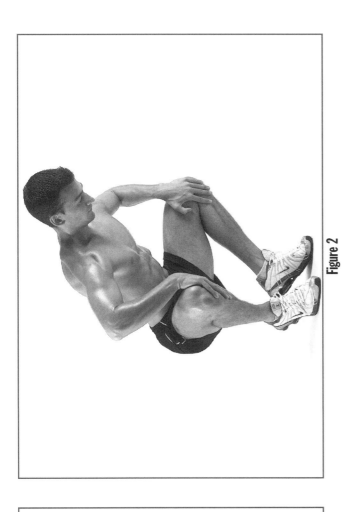

Figure 2

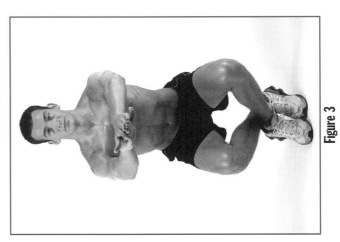

Figure 3

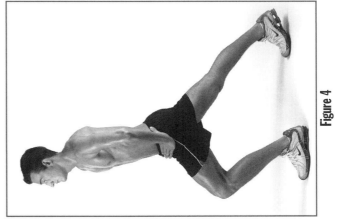

Figure 4

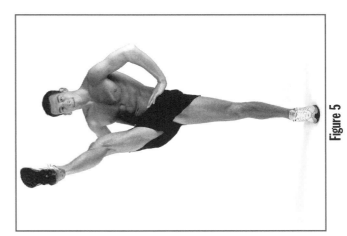

Figure 5

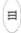

POWERFLEX
SHOULDERS

FLEXERCISE
THE·TOTAL·BODY·WORKOUT

SHOULDERS WORKOUT

You can have well-rounded, powerful, healthy shoulders without using equipment, weights, pulleys, or machines. Just do five Flexercises for 20 minutes a day.

Flexercise™ for Well-Rounded, Powerful, Healthy Shoulders

It's no accident that when people are feeling burdened, they say they're carrying the weight of the world on their shoulders. We see broad, powerful shoulders and think of heroes—those with the strength to bear heavy burdens confidently and successfully, to defend themselves and protect and nurture others.

Perhaps the most inspiring shoulders in the animal kingdom belong to the gorilla. Its massively broad, thick shoulders reflect the frightening strength and power it displays when defending its territory. Yet when the danger has passed, the gorilla bears its young on those same shoulders as it travels and eats. The sight of such a small, fragile being clinging to the neck of such a huge, powerful one can arouse tenderness in any human parent.

The Flexercises in this Workout not only imitate the gorilla's movements, but also those of the rhinoceros and the cougar. Whatever your burdens, and for whomever you bear them, let these Flexercises help you develop shoulders ready to defend, nurture, and inspire.

Ready? Let's Flexercise™!

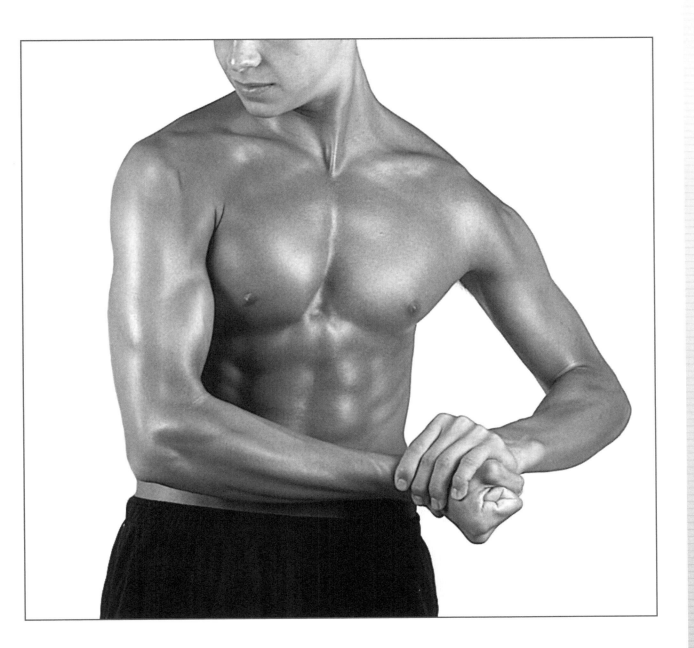

#1 GORILLA FLEX II

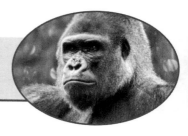

This Flexercise™ is similar to a gorilla using its fist to push something away.

Sit or stand. Bend your right arm at the elbow until your forearm is parallel to the floor. Make a fist with your right hand and place your left palm over your fist. Slowly and smoothly push your right fist forward while resisting with the left hand. Return to the starting position and repeat. Reverse the movement to work your left shoulder.

LEVEL THREE: 80 repetitions (40 per side)
LEVEL TWO: 40 repetitions
LEVEL ONE: 20 repetitions

As with all Flexercises, don't be in a hurry to add repetitions. Remember that your success with Flexercise™ depends more on the amount of tension you use than on the number of repetitions you do. Make each repetition perfect!

SHOULDERS

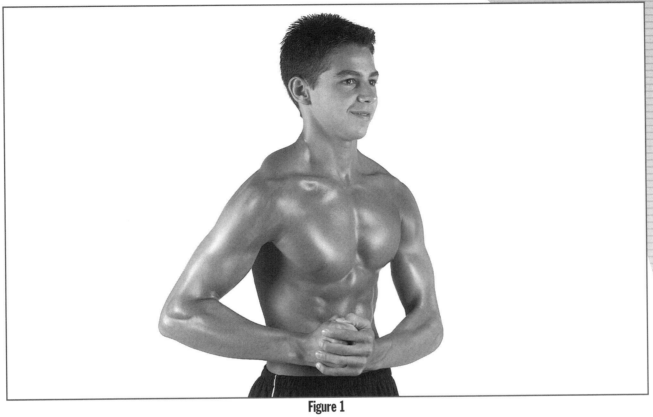

Figure 1

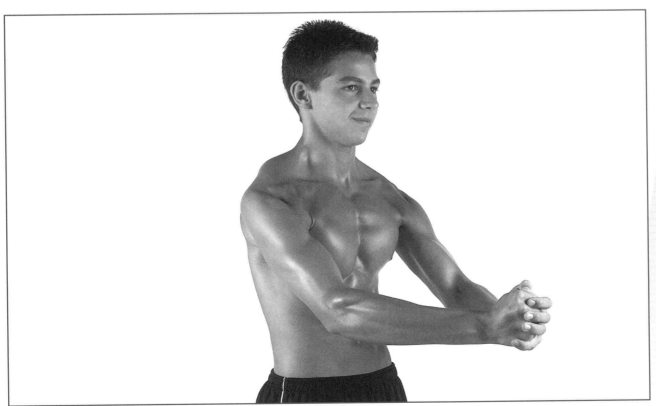

Figure 2

#2 GORILLA FLEX III

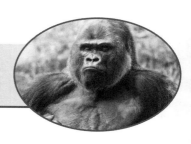

This Flexercise™ simulates the way the gorilla pulls itself across and up a tree branch as it climbs.

Sit or stand. Raise your left elbow until you're holding it across your chest. Place the palm of your right hand under your left elbow. Slowly and smoothly pull your elbow back down to your left side as you resist with your right hand. Return to the starting position and repeat. Reverse the movement to work your right shoulder.

LEVEL THREE: 60 repetitions (30 per side)
LEVEL TWO: 40 repetitions
LEVEL ONE: 20 repetitions

The muscles of the front, middle, and rear shoulder allow you to move your arms up, down, and around. Developing strong, impressive shoulders means developing all of these muscles. This Flexercise™ works the rear shoulder muscles.

SHOULDERS

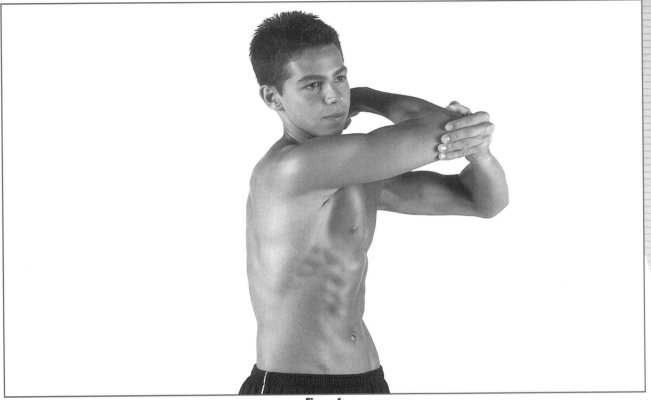

Figure 1

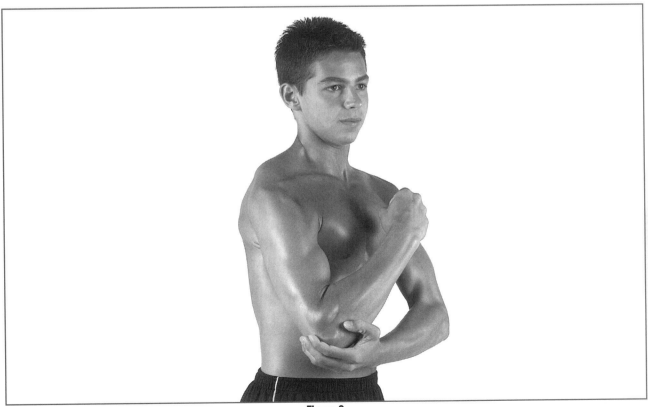

Figure 2

POWERFLEX

#3 RHINO FLEX I

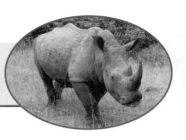

The rhinoceros has such huge shoulders, it seems as though it doesn't have a neck! Thanks to the immense muscles along the tops of its shoulders, the bulky rhino can pull its legs through deep, sucking mud. Your next Flexercise™ simulates that movement.

Sit or stand. With your left hand, reach behind your back and grasp your right wrist. Slowly and smoothly, raise your right shoulder as high as you can, resisting with your left hand. Return to the starting position and repeat. Reverse the movement to work your left shoulder.

> **LEVEL THREE:** 60 repetitions (30 per side)
> **LEVEL TWO:** 40 repetitions
> **LEVEL ONE:** 20 repetitions

SHOULDERS

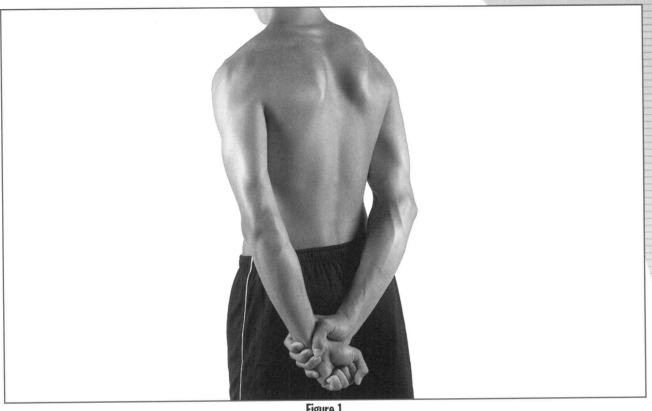

Figure 1

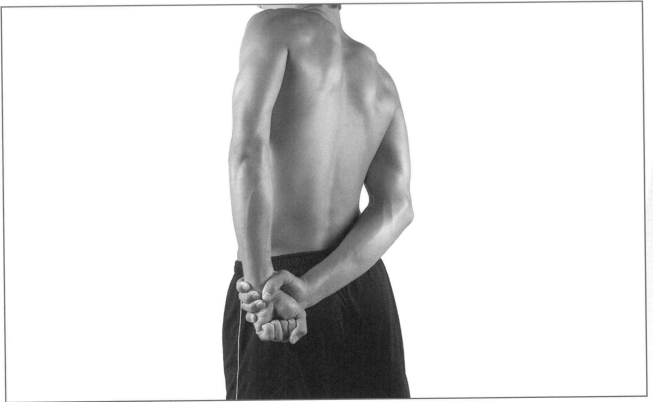

Figure 2

#4 COUGAR FLEX I

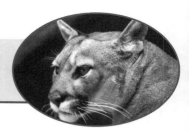

The cougar is a fearsome predator, moving quietly, then striking with deadly force. Its powerful shoulders allow it to overpower its prey and to wield its sharp claws with pinpoint control. This Flexercise™ simulates that striking movement. It's excellent for developing the middle shoulder muscles.

Sit or stand. Raise your right arm across your body just beneath chest level. Your right palm should be facing down. With your left hand, grasp your right wrist. Slowly and smoothly push your right arm up and out while resisting with your left hand. Return to the starting position and repeat. Reverse the movement to work your left shoulder.

LEVEL THREE: 80 repetitions (40 per side)
LEVEL TWO: 40 repetitions
LEVEL ONE: 20 repetitions

SHOULDERS

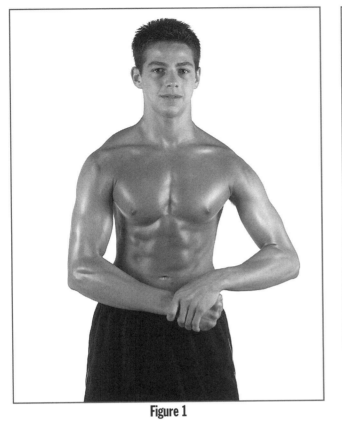

Figure 1

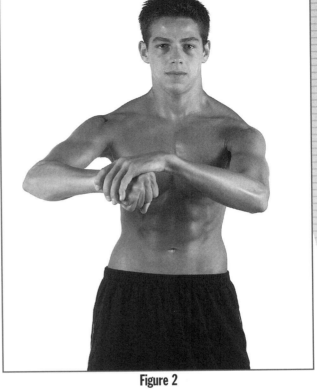

Figure 2

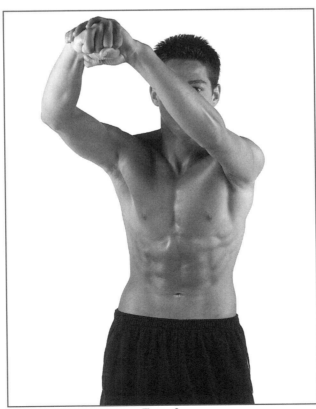

Figure 3

#5 COUGAR FLEX II

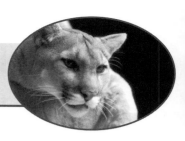

After taking its prey, the cougar tears its flesh and begins to feed. The last Flexercise™ of this workout simulates that tearing movement—raw power at its max.

Sit or stand. Raise your left arm across your stomach. Your left palm should be facing up. With your right hand, grasp your left wrist. Slowly and smoothly pull your left hand back toward your left side while resisting with your right hand. Return to the starting position and repeat. Reverse the movement to work your right shoulder.

LEVEL THREE: 60 repetitions (30 per side)
LEVEL TWO: 40 repetitions
LEVEL ONE: 20 repetitions

Practice these five Flexercises with consistency, determination, and patience, and reap the rewards: shoulders with the strength to defend, nurture, and inspire, and the confidence that goes with them.

SHOULDERS

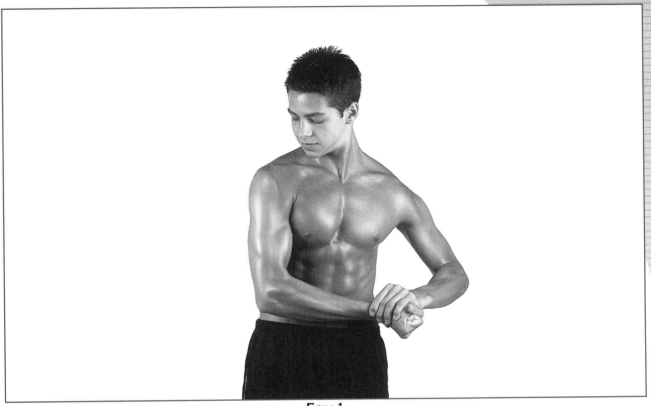

Figure 1

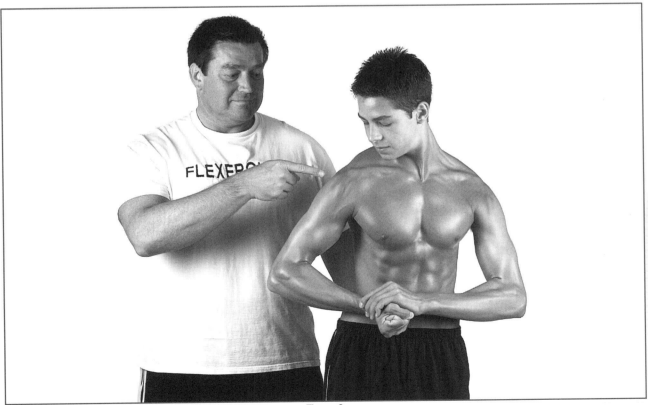

Figure 2

POWERFLEX

SHOULDER EXERCISES

GORILLA FLEX II figure 1

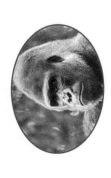

GORILLA FLEX III figure 2

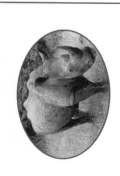

RHINO FLEX I figure 3

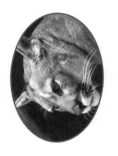

COUGAR FLEX I figure 4

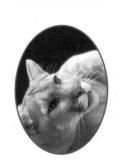

COUGAR FLEX II figure 5

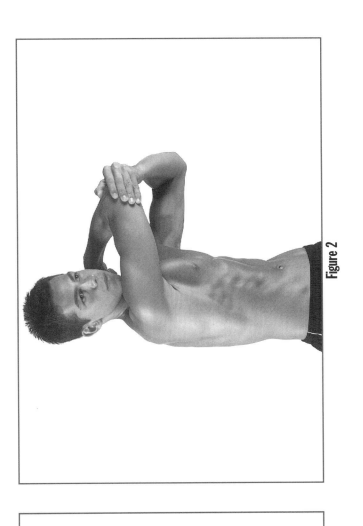

Figure 1

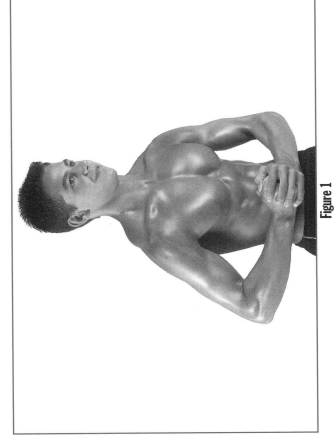

Figure 2

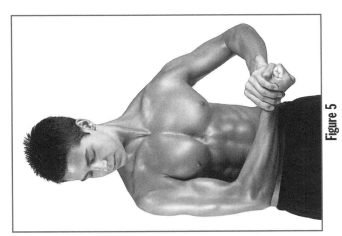

Figure 5

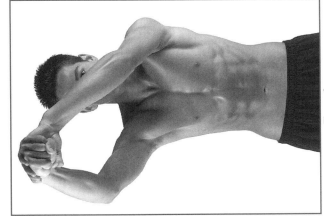

Figure 4

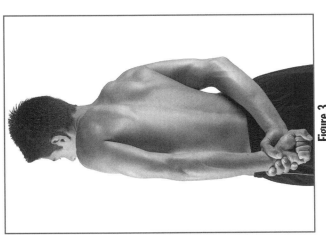

Figure 3

POWERFLEX
ARMS

FLEXERCISE
THE·TOTAL·BODY·WORKOUT

ARMS WORKOUT

You can have strong, muscular, well-shaped, awesome arms without using equipment, weights, pulleys, or machines. Just do five Flexercises for 20 minutes a day.

Flexercise™ for Strong, Muscular, Well-Defined Arms

Why does the gorilla flex and display its huge arms when confronting a rival gorilla? Why do many NFL offensive linemen leave their arms bare when they play in frigid winter weather? Because a pair of well-muscled arms—with bulging biceps in front, horseshoe-shaped triceps behind, and thickly corded forearms beneath—is an impressive, intimidating sight. Whether your goal is to protect your "turf" (or your quarterback) or to attract a mate, big arms are the symbol of strength and authority.

If you've practiced the earlier workouts with consistency, determination, and patience, your arms are already stronger, bigger, and more muscular than they were, thanks to all the indirect work you gave them when you were Flexercising your chest, back, legs, and shoulders. Now that you've built a strong foundation, the following five Flexercises will work your arms directly—and help you build the biceps, triceps, and forearms you've always wanted.

The Flexercises in this Workout imitate the movements of the gorilla, lion, tiger, and jaguar, five creatures who climb with amazing ease and strike with overwhelming force.

All set? Time to Flexercise™!

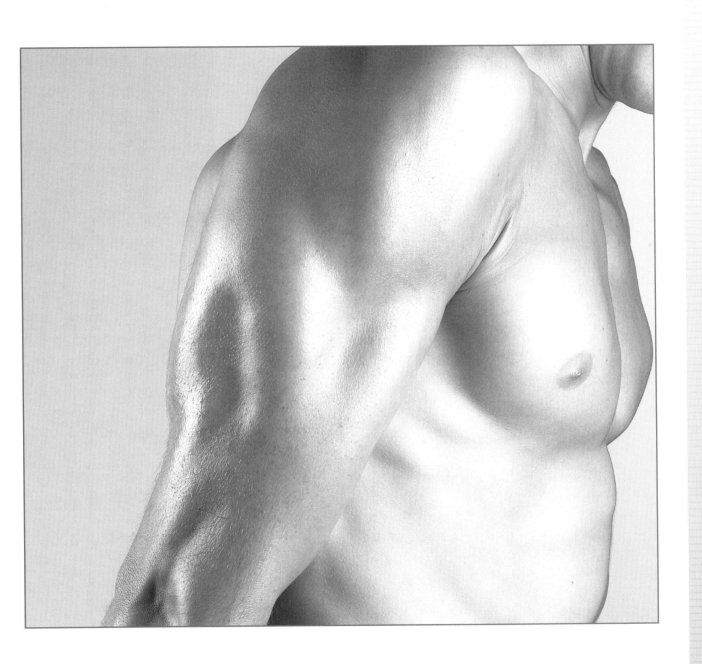

#1 GORILLA FLEX IV

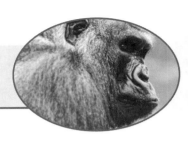

The gorilla has inspired five of the Flexercises in this course. You did the first one in the Chest Workout, the second and third ones in the Arm workout, and here's number four.

To build impressive arms, it's important to work the biceps, triceps, and forearms from many different angles. This unique Flexercise™ works the biceps from two angles.

Part One: sit or stand, with your right arm hanging at your side and your right hand palm up. With your left hand, grasp your right wrist. Slowly and smoothly bend your right elbow and pull your right hand toward your shoulder as you resist with your left hand. Lower your right hand and repeat. Reverse the movement to work your left arm.

Part Two: same starting position as Part One. Reach behind your back with your left hand and grasp your right wrist. Slowly and smoothly, bend your right elbow and pull your right hand toward your shoulder as you resist with your left hand. Lower your right hand and repeat. Reverse the movement to work your left arm.

LEVEL THREE: 60 repetitions (15 per arm for both Parts)
LEVEL TWO: 40 repetitions
LEVEL ONE: 20 repetitions

If you have short arms and/or tight shoulders, you may find Part Two difficult to do. Try to let the elbow of the working arm move back and pull your hand toward your armpit as far as you can without straining.

ARMS

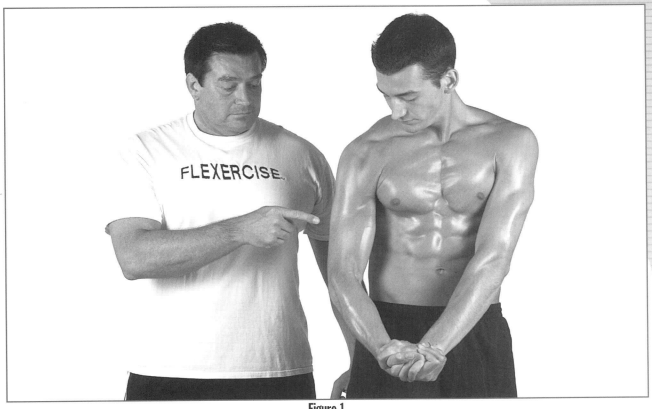

Figure 1

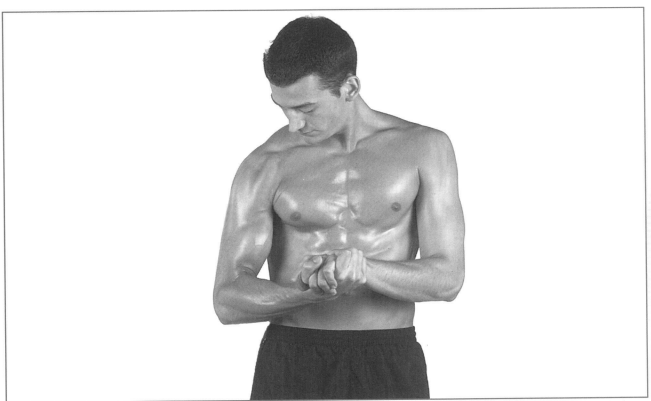

Figure 2

#2 LION FLEX I

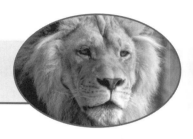

The lion's incredible speed and strength allow it to overcome animals much larger than itself, like the elephant and the water buffalo. Your next Flexercise™ (for the triceps) simulates the way the lion reaches out to slash its prey.

Sit or stand, with your right arm hanging at your side. Make a fist with your right hand. Bend your right elbow and pull your right hand toward your shoulder. With your left hand, grasp your right fist from beneath. Keeping your right elbow close to your side, slowly and smoothly push your right hand down and out as you resist with your left hand. Raise your right hand and repeat. Reverse the movement to work your left arm.

LEVEL THREE: 60 repetitions (30 per side)
LEVEL TWO: 40 repetitions
LEVEL ONE: 20 repetitions

ARMS

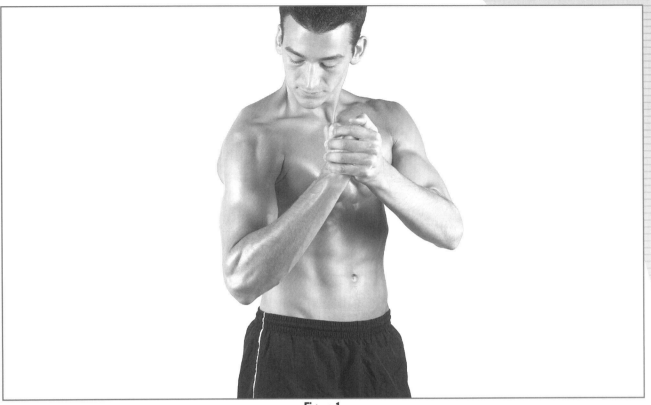

Figure 1

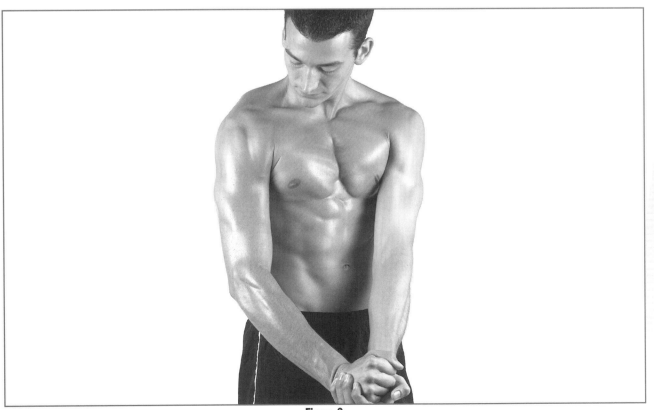

Figure 2

#3 TIGER FLEX I

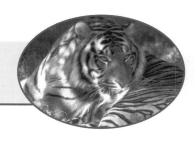

Like the lion, the tiger is feared for its lightning-fast strikes and razor-sharp claws. Similar to Lion Flex I, this next Flexercise™ also works the triceps, but from a different angle.

Sit or stand. Raise your right arm and hold it across your chest. With your left hand, grasp the back of your right wrist. Keeping your right upper arm close to your side, slowly and smoothly push your right forearm up and out while resisting with your left hand. Return to the starting position and repeat. Reverse the movement to work your left arm.

LEVEL THREE: 40 repetitions (20 per side)
LEVEL TWO: 20 repetitions
LEVEL ONE: 10 repetitions

ARMS

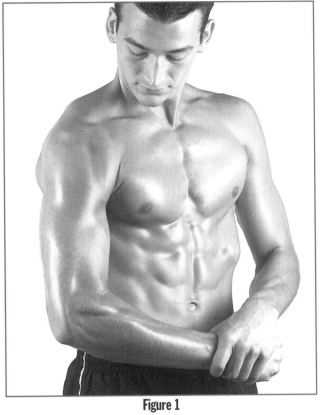

Figure 1

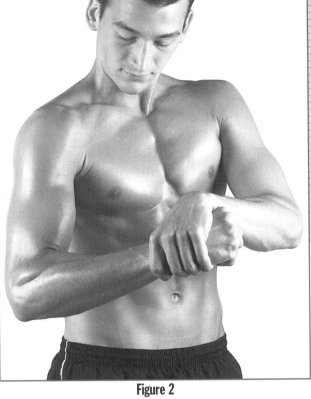

Figure 2

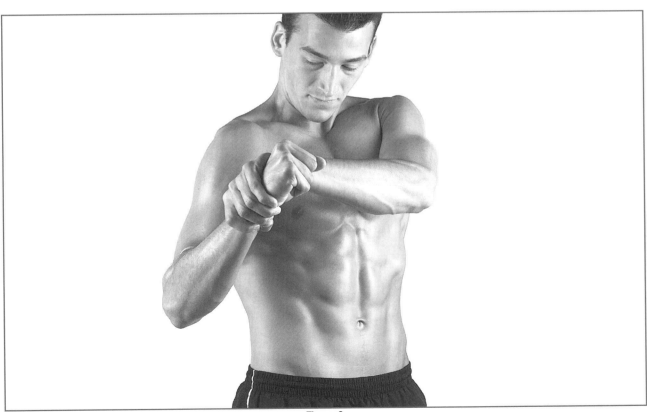

Figure 3

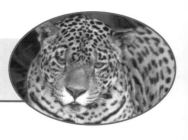

#4 JAGUAR FLEX I

It's amazing to watch slow-motion film of a running jaguar. With every stride, the jaguar pulls itself forward, then stretches its legs, grasps the ground with its feet, and pulls again. This Flexercise™ simulates these movements and works the biceps, triceps, and forearms all at once.

Sit or stand, with your arms hanging at your sides. With your thumbs facing forward, make your hands into tight fists. Slowly and smoothly, bend both of your arms at the elbows and twist your fists until your palms are facing the tops of your shoulders (as though you're a bodybuilder doing a "double biceps" pose). Lower your arms slowly and smoothly. When you return to the starting position, push back on your arms (as though you're trying to bend them backward at the elbows) for a second or two. Repeat.

> **LEVEL THREE:** 20 repetitions
> **LEVEL TWO:** 10 repetitions
> **LEVEL ONE:** 5 repetitions

Keep your fists tight and feel the tension in your forearms. As you raise your fists, feel the tension in your biceps. As you lower your fists and push back on your arms, feel the tension in your triceps. Remember that developing your body with Flexercise™ has more to do with tension than with repetition.

ARMS

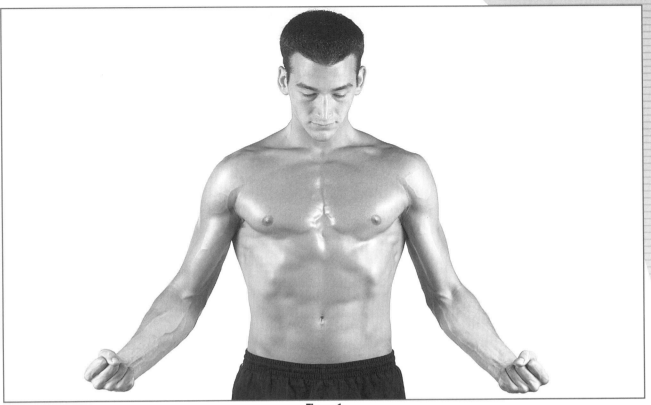

Figure 1

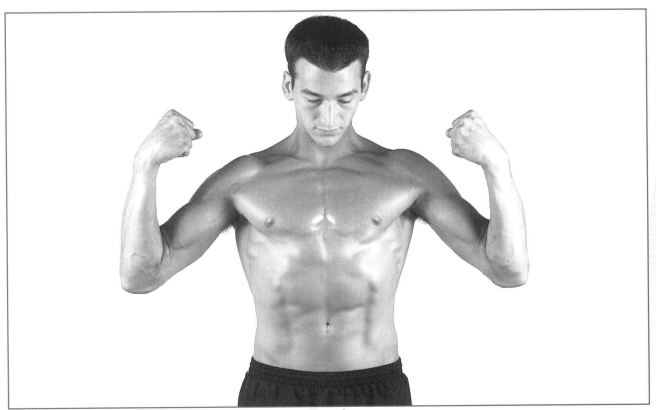

Figure 3

#5 GORILLA FLEX V

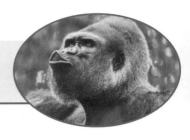

This Gorilla Flex is a fine all-in-one Flexercise™ for your biceps, triceps, and forearms.

Part One: sit or stand, with your arms hanging at your sides. Your hands should be open with the palms facing your sides. Push back on your arms (as you did for Jaguar Flex I) for a second or two. Now shake the tension out of your arms and relax for a few moments.

Part Two: next, make a fist with your right hand. Bend your right arm at the elbow and twist your fist until your palm is facing the top of your right shoulder (as you did with both arms for Jaguar Flex I). Hold this position for a second or two, then relax your right arm.

Part Three: same as for Part Two, but reverse the movement to work your left arm.

One cycle through all three parts counts as one repetition.

> **LEVEL THREE:** 20 repetitions
> **LEVEL TWO:** 10 repetitions
> **LEVEL ONE:** 5 repetitions

There you go, friend—a complete Flexercise™ Workout for building arms that mean business. Thanks to the strong foundation you've built through practicing the previous Workouts, adding these concentrated Flexercises to your routine will add muscle to your arms very quickly. As always, emphasize tension when you Flexercise™—see and feel your muscles as they work, and imagine them gaining the strength, size, and shape you're seeking. After all, what the mind believes, the body will achieve!

ARMS

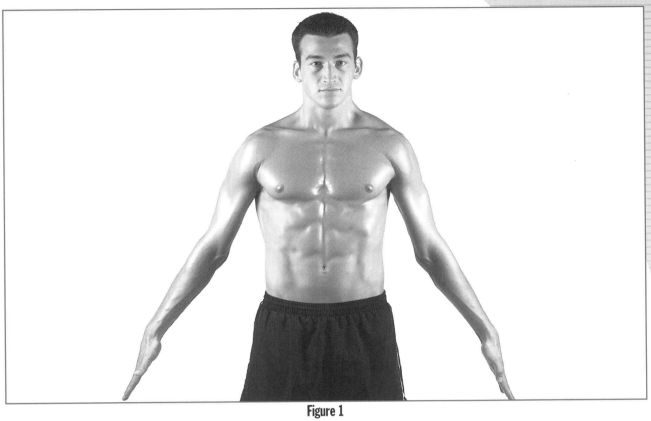

Figure 1

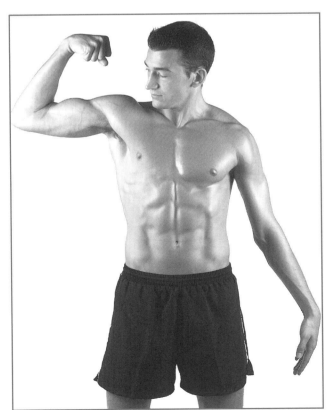

Figure 2

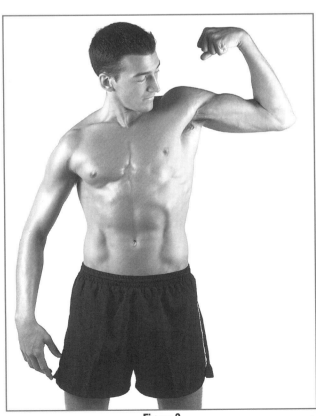

Figure 3

ARM EXERCISES

GORILLA FLEX IV — figure 1

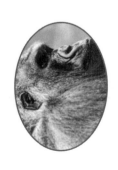

LION FLEX I — figure 2

TIGER FLEX I — figure 3

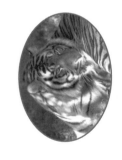

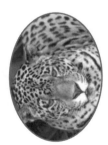

JAGUAR FLEX I — figure 4

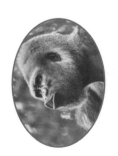

GORILLA FLEX V — figure 5

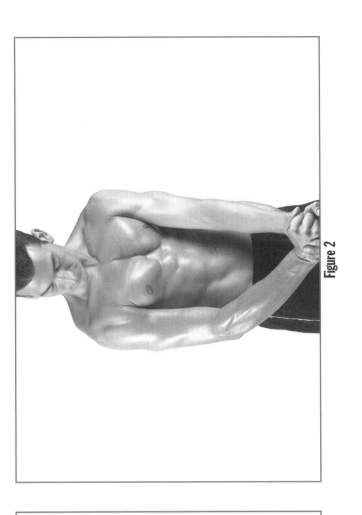

Figure 2

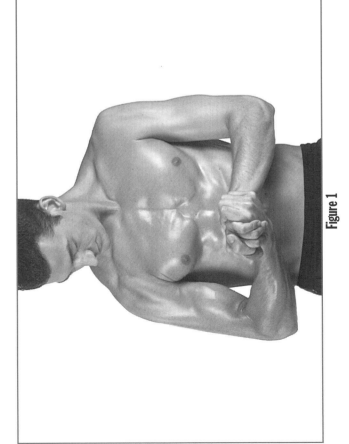

Figure 1

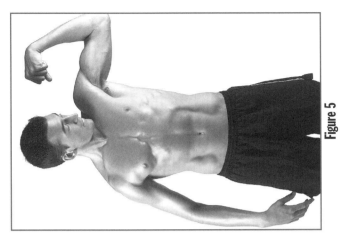

Figure 5

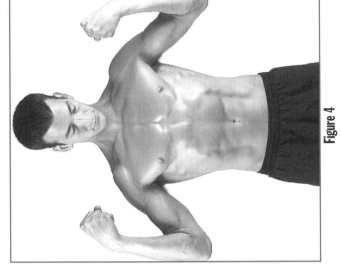

Figure 4

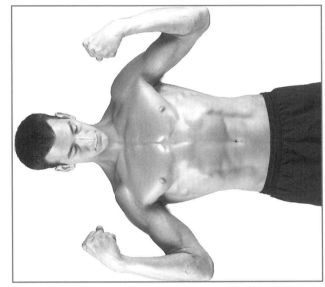

Figure 3

POWERFLEX
SPEED, ENERGY
and ENDURANCE

FLEXERCISE
THE·TOTAL·BODY·WORKOUT

SPEED, ENERGY and ENDURANCE WORKOUT

You can have speed, energy, and endurance without using equipment, weights, pulleys, or machines. Just do five Flexercises for 20 minutes a day.

Flexercise™ for Speed, Energy, and Endurance

In the animal kingdom, "show" means "go." That is, creatures can actually do everything they look like they can do. The stocky, short-legged mule can actually haul huge loads up and over mountain passes. The lean, sinewy cheetah can actually accelerate to 67 miles per hour in three seconds flat. The massively muscular bear can actually tear a door off its hinges with one paw.

If you've practiced the last eight Workouts with consistency, determination, and patience, you've transformed your "show." The Chest Workout helped you deepen your chest. The Back Workout helped you develop a V-shaped upper body. The Shoulder and Arm Workouts helped you broaden your shoulders and shape your arms.

For most of this course, you've Flexercised no more than two parts of your body on any given day. Now, before you graduate, you're ready for a Workout that will work your whole body, all at once. The following Workout begins and ends with a stretch and challenges you to climb, dash, and trot. These activities will teach your body how to coordinate and use the strength and fitness you've already developed and will build your speed, energy, and endurance. Here's where you add more "go" to your "show!"

On your mark! Get set! Flexercise!

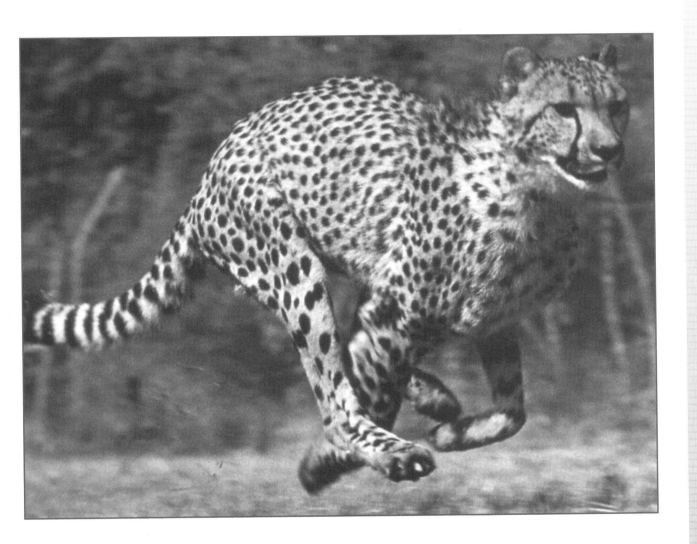

#1 CHEETAH FLEX I

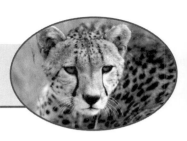

Cats…shred…everything. It doesn't matter whether they're super-predators, such as lions, tigers, or cheetahs, or tabby housecats that hide when the doorbell rings. They reach forward with their front paws, grab the grass (or carpet or couch), pull back, and stretch their back and legs. They don't do it to be nasty, but to strengthen their muscles and stay limber—it's their version of Flexercise™! This first Flexercise™ imitates that movement (without trashing the furniture).

Stand with your feet shoulder-width apart and your hands on your hips. Keeping your legs straight, bend forward slowly and smoothly as far as you can without straining. With your right hand, try to touch the floor in front of your left foot. Return to the starting position, then bend forward again. With your left hand, try to touch the floor in front of your right foot. Return to the starting position and repeat.

LEVEL THREE: 100 repetitions (50 per side)
LEVEL TWO: 50 repetitions
LEVEL ONE: 30 repetitions

Don't worry if you can't touch the floor at first, or even your ankle. If you don't feel comfortable reaching below your knee, that's fine—start where you are. Never, ever strain! Practice this Flexercise™ with consistency, determination, and patience, and see how quickly your flexibility and endurance improve.

SPEED, ENERGY, & ENDURANCE

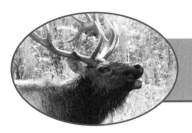

#2 ELK CLIMB

I love to spend time in the high mountains, where the thin air forces some visitors to pant, even when they're standing still. Thanks to regular Flexercise™, I have the strength, energy, and endurance to hike and climb at high altitudes. I feel blessed that I can climb high enough to see and appreciate sights people can't see from their cars—such as a half-ton bull elk bounding up a steep slope at 10,000 feet as easily as I'd walk through the meadow far below.

Fortunately, you don't need a mountain to build the fitness to climb one. Just find some stairs. A set of stadium steps or the stairs at an office or apartment building would be ideal, but you can get the same results climbing the stairs in your home.

Once you've found some stairs, run up and down them if you can, but if that's a strain, it's fine to walk. Don't try to move so fast that you stumble or can't get your breath. This Flexercise™ will build your agility and endurance quickly. One trip up and down counts as one repetition.

> **LEVEL THREE:** 20 repetitions
> **LEVEL TWO:** 10 repetitions
> **LEVEL ONE:** 5 repetitions

NOTE: These are general guidelines only. The longer your set of stairs is, the fewer repetitions you'll need.

#3 CHEETAH DASH

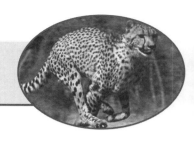

The thoroughbred horse and the greyhound are celebrated for their speed, but Mother Nature's fastest sprinter—hands down—is the cheetah. When chasing its prey, the cheetah can accelerate to highway speed limits more quickly than most cars.

You'll probably never have to chase down your supper. But if you're an athlete, you know that winning often depends on speed. It's the difference between getting the takedown and being taken down by your opponent. The difference between catching the touchdown pass and watching it sail through the end zone, just beyond your reach.

First, pace off and mark a 40-yard stretch of grass (at a park or schoolyard or on your own lawn) or track (at a school athletic field) or pavement (on a lightly-traveled street or sidewalk). Now, sprint the distance. Lift your knees and pump your arms, and don't let up until you've run through your finish line. Rest for 15 seconds (either timed with a stopwatch or counted to yourself), then sprint back to your starting point.

> **LEVEL THREE:** 10 repetitions
> **LEVEL TWO:** 7 repetitions
> **LEVEL ONE:** 5 repetitions

Even if you're not an athlete, practicing this Flexercise™ can give you a burst of speed to catch a bus or cross a busy street. It can help you look better, too. Research has shown that sprinting not only burns fat more effectively than long distance running but that it builds muscle, too.

If you're new to sprinting, don't run all out at first—you don't want to pull a muscle. Feel free to rest for more than 15 seconds between repetitions, if you need to. In time, you won't need so much rest. Don't strain! If you'd rather not sprint, that's okay—fast walking works just fine. And you don't need grass, track, or pavement—a large room will do.

SPEED, ENERGY, & ENDURANCE

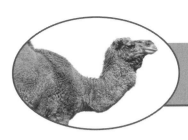

#4 CAMEL TROT

Imagine that a cheetah and a camel decide to run a 200-mile race through the desert. The cheetah will probably jump to a quick lead. But long after the cheetah will have given up, worn out by the distance and the heat, the camel will still be striding slowly and steadily—almost rolling—over the sand to victory.

The moral of the story: speed is a valuable trait, whether you're an animal, an athlete, or an accountant. But for complete health and fitness, a human needs endurance, too. After all, some days seem like a series of all-out dashes and others feel like slow-motion marathons. Practicing the Camel Trot can give you the endurance to finish even your longest days with energy to spare.

First, measure out a one-mile stretch of grass, track, or sidewalk. If you ran the Cheetah Dash on an outdoor track, you can Camel Trot there, too—a mile equals about four laps. Then, slowly and smoothly jog the distance. The object isn't to break the four-minute mile, but to maintain a slow, steady rhythm. Try to jog like the camel: roll your feet along heel-to-toe instead of slapping them down. Pounding the ground wastes energy and can cause injuries.

REMEMBER: Flexercise™ is about training, not straining!

If running doesn't feel comfortable for you, it's no problem. Walk the distance instead, as briskly as you can without straining. Brisk walking is a healing, energizing activity—that's why doctors recommend it so highly, even for heart patients. For humans, walking is the most natural exercise there is. Give yourself the chance to move. And to enjoy moving!

#5 CHEETAH FLEX II

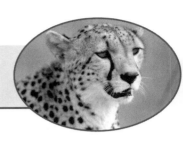

Now that you've climbed, dashed, and trotted, your muscles and joints are well warmed up. This last Flexercise™ is similar to Cheetah Flex I and will stretch your legs, hips, and back to help prevent post-workout stiffness and cramping.

Stand with your feet together and your hands on your hips. Keeping your legs straight, bend forward slowly and smoothly as far as you can without straining. With both hands, try to touch the floor in front of your feet. Return to the starting position and repeat.

> **LEVEL THREE:** 20 repetitions
> **LEVEL TWO:** 10 repetitions
> **LEVEL ONE:** 5 repetitions

Don't worry if you can't reach your feet, or even your ankles. Don't bend over farther than you can comfortably. In time, your flexibility will improve. Remember: Flexercise™ isn't a contest. It's supposed to feel good!

There you go, friend—the last Workout in this Flexercise™ course. Practice it with consistency, determination, and patience, and feel the new "Go"—the new speed, energy, and endurance—in your "Show."

SPEED, ENERGY, & ENDURANCE

A FINAL WORD

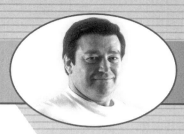

Dear Friend,

Once again, think about where you've come from and where you are. And where you're going.

If you've followed the Workout rotation I recommended earlier in this course, you've been Flexercising for eight weeks. During that time, you've learned and practiced 45 Flexercises—none requiring special equipment, only your own consistency, determination, and patience. Your courage in choosing to build a stronger, healthier, more attractive body, and your imagination in seeing and feeling that body develop, has transformed not just your body, but transformed you! You've seen and felt what it is to work toward a goal and achieve it. What advantage you've taken of this opportunity! What gifts you've given yourself!

NOW, WHAT'S NEXT?

The wild animals, whose pulling, pushing, stretching, and running inspired Flexercise™, stay healthy and fit for as long as they live. And with Flexercise™, you can, too. Now that you've "graduated," feel free to experiment. Create your own Flexercise™ Workouts, using the ideas in the Introduction to guide you. Now that you've developed your "mind-muscle connection," you can even invent your own Flexercises! Keep studying the ways you move, and the ways animals move. You've given yourself the tools to be your own best personal trainer. Just remember that managing tension, not doing endless repetitions, is the key.

Friend, the gifts you've earned can and should be yours for life. But gifts such as yours become even more valuable when shared with others. You decided what you wanted to change, and you've become—and are becoming—that change, that person. You've given yourself the permission to be better, and being better has become a habit. Through your appearance, and through your thoughts, words, and deeds, you can give others permission to be better, too. To become their best selves. And to create a more healthy, positive, hopeful world for themselves, and all of us, to live in. Make this your practice, too. Just like Flexercising!

I want to give you a diploma recognizing your achievement—something you can frame and look at to remind yourself of where you've come from, where you are, and where you're going. I hope you'll fill out the application on the following page and return it to me. If you like, send me a few words about your experience with Flexercise™. It would be my privilege to rejoice with you in your success.

Thank you for allowing me to share this course with you, and for allowing me to help you begin to build the body—and life—you were always meant to have.

Your Friend,

Jim Forystek

Jim Forystek
Creator, Flexercise™

QUESTION & ANSWERS

1. Why do Flexercise™ when I could be lifting weights instead?

It seems as though most veteran weightlifters suffer from what my friend John Peterson calls "Busted-Up Weightlifter's Syndrome." I've been approached by many, many weightlifters who are dealing with chronic physical problems, including deteriorated discs and joints, torn cartilage, torn ligaments, and torn muscles. They've got bad backs, elbows, shoulders, hips, and knees. And unfortunately, many have learned to live with chronic pain.

Early on in a weightlifting workout, the muscles are still fresh enough to do the work of moving the weight. But after a few sets, once the muscles become fatigued, they're less able to support and move the weight. This means the joints, tendons, and ligaments have to do it: a surefire recipe for injury. Over time, heavy weightlifting compresses the spine, squeezing the spinal fluid out of the discs that separate the vertebrae. When there's no padding left to separate the discs, you're left with bone rubbing against bone. And pain.

Unlike weightlifting, Flexercise™ doesn't stress the spine, joints, and connective tissue with added weight. Instead, Flexercise™ uses the body's own energy to provide resistance. It turns the body's natural movements—stretching, pulling, pushing, and flexing—into safe, healthful tools for developing strength, flexibility, and vitality.

If you can bench press 400 pounds plus, you're very, very strong. But if your shoulders are so stiff and sore that you can't scratch your back between the shoulder blades, Flexercise™ can help you improve your flexibility, heal your injuries, and get your body back.

2. What's the advantage of Flexercise™ over running and other forms of aerobic exercise?

"Aerobic" means "with oxygen," and it's essential that you breathe deeply and regularly while doing your Flexercises. Doing this will fill your muscles with the fresh, oxygen-rich blood that muscles need to grow and develop.

Actually, all of the Flexercises in this course are aerobic, except for one: The Cheetah Dash. This one isn't aerobic because it involves sprinting—running so fast that the body can't eliminate waste products from the muscles fast enough to continue for very long. For complete health and fitness, it's important to practice both non-aerobic activities, such as sprinting, and aerobic ones, such as most of the Flexercises.

Sprinting and jogging are excellent. That's why, along with the Cheetah Dash, this course also includes the Camel Trot. However, running alone isn't enough to build complete fitness. And running long distances (longer than five miles) can, over time, cause chronic overuse injuries to the feet, ankles, knees, hips, and back similar to "Busted-Up Weightlifter's Syndrome."

Folks whose only exercise is running long distances, or taking step aerobics or "spinning" classes, usually look healthy when they're fully clothed. But when they strip down, the picture often changes. Because their routines don't include muscle-building exercises, they may have skinny arms, narrow shoulders, and sunken chests. Maybe even flabby abs.

If you run long distances, you owe it to your long-term health to supplement your running with a low-impact, joint-friendly strength training program such as Flexercise™. Combining long distance running and Flexercise™ won't give you massive muscles, but it will improve your "finishing kick" and help you recover from long runs more quickly. And you'll look good in shorts and a t-shirt, too!

3. Why do Flexercise™ instead of working out at a gym or a health/fitness club?

If you join a health club, you're paying constantly—to be taught how to use the exercise equipment, then to continue to use it. You pay for that equipment to be maintained and sanitized regularly. And for all the extras, such as juice bars and cable TV, whether you use or want them or not.

If you've got a tight schedule, working out at a health club means finding time to drive to the club, find a parking place, change clothes, and stand in line to use the equipment—whether the equipment has been sanitized or not.

This Flexercise™ course provides much better value for your money. It's like an owner's manual for the human body, showing you how to use your own energy and ability to build strength, health, and vitality. You can Flexercise™ wherever you are, whenever it's convenient. You can listen to your favorite music or watch your favorite TV show. You only pay for it once. But with consistency, determination, and patience, your investment will pay for itself over and over again.

4. Why Flexercise™ instead of using one of those home gym machines?

Consider the cost. Many of those treadmills, exercycles, ski machines, and weight machines cost hundreds—or thousands—of dollars. And once the maintenance contract runs out—if you bought one—repair bills add to your cost.

Exercise machines are not only expensive, but they can be dangerous, too. Seats and pins break, benches collapse, and bands snap—sometimes causing serious injuries. Thousands of these contraptions have been recalled by their manufacturers due to mechanical breakdowns (and lawsuits). On TV they always work perfectly and take up minimal floor space. But once they're delivered and set up, they're often bigger than they appear on TV. And more difficult to use.

All these reasons explain why so many exercise machines become big, expensive racks for drying clothes, and why so many owners give up and try to sell them, hoping to get back even a fraction of their investment.

Flexercise™ is a far better value. You're paying for information, not for big, expensive, complicated gadgets. You only pay for it once, and it's as portable as you are. You can Flexercise™ whenever it's convenient. And best of all, Flexercise™ teaches you how to get the most out of the most brilliantly designed, incredibly functional machine you'll ever use: your own body.

5. How fit do I have to be before I can do Flexercise™?

Whether you're already fit from other activities or have never exercised in your life, Flexercise™ lets you start where you are and can help you reach your fitness goals, whatever they are. With consistency, determination, and patience, you can build huge, bulging muscles and massive strength, like a gorilla, or lean, sculpted muscles with explosive power, like a panther. The more tension you use and the higher the number of repetitions you do, the bigger your muscles will grow. Achieving your fitness goals won't always be easy. But with Flexercise™, you have the tools to make it simple.

6. What makes Flexercise™ better than other exercise or fitness courses?

Flexercise™ doesn't rely on expensive, unreliable machines to achieve results. Instead, Flexercise™ is about information. This course gives you complete instructions, explaining and illustrating how to perform each Flexercise™, along with instructions for rotating your Workouts to achieve the quickest results possible.

Flexercise™ gives you room to be creative, too. With 45 Flexercises to choose from, it's simple to create workouts that let you focus on a particular body part. And if you crave variety, you can build five completely different, full-body workouts of your own and never do the same Flexercise™ twice! Flexercise™ works, because it works for you.

A Word From
Dr. Dwight Tamanaha

As a holistic consultant and personal trainer and a public speaker on impact-overexertion trauma for PERformance Enterprises International, I am successfully working with amateur and professional explosive strength athletes. I find the Flexercise™ workout program to be one of the most effective and powerful ways to build massive amounts of muscle with maximum results in so little time! Building the normally weaker upper body region is crucial for protection against impact-overexertion trauma. The accompaniment of breathing with these exercises pushes oxygen deep into the tissues being exercised.

Dr. Dwight Tamanaha,
Doctor of Chiropractic
Certified Chiropractic Sports Physician

Dr. Tamanaha is a record-holding Olympic weightlifter in his age and weight class. A former All-American and National Champion, he is published in the *Southern Medical Journal,* in a medical textbook, and in the world almanac.

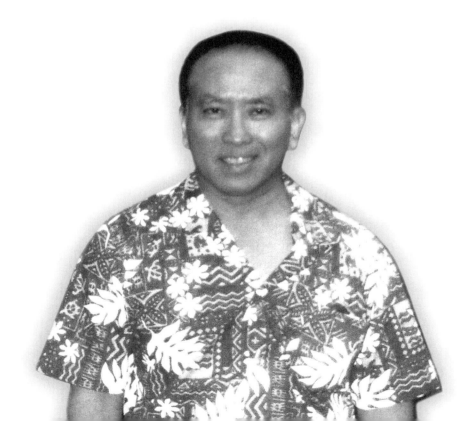

From JOHN & WENDIE

ANYTIME. ANYWHERE. TOTAL STRENGTH & FITNESS FOR MEN & WOMEN.

Imagine a complete strength and fitness program that slims, shapes, and sculpts your entire body in just 20 minutes a day. A program you can do anytime and virtually anywhere. A program so complete it requires no gym and no exercise equipment. Best of all, a program that covers every muscle group from your neck to your toes and delivers visible results in as little as 3 weeks.

Using the revolutionary Transformetrics™ Training System that utilizes time-tested body sculpting techniques along with high-tension Isometrics that literally allow you to become your own gym, *The Miracle Seven* offers:

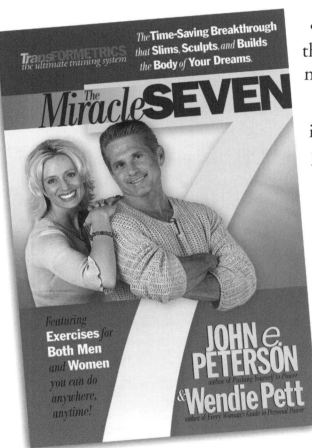

• A 20-minute per day weekly plan that sculpts the entire body to its own natural perfection.

• Detailed day-by-day exercise instruction, fully illustrated with photos that show each and every exercise.

• A special "speed it up" program that accelerates fat-burning results for those who want to see their results yesterday.

• A comprehensive nutrition plan that allows you to lose body fat faster than you gained it while providing easy to follow guidelines for eating healthy.

• The exhilaration that comes from knowing that you have complete control over your body, your life, and your destiny!

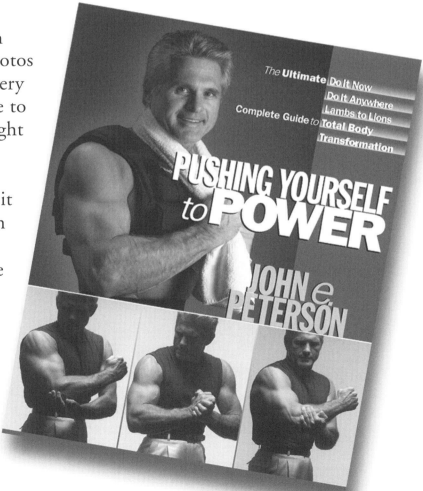

Receive Your Own Flexercise™ Certificate of Achievement,

Signed Personally by the Creator of Flexercise™, Jim Forystek

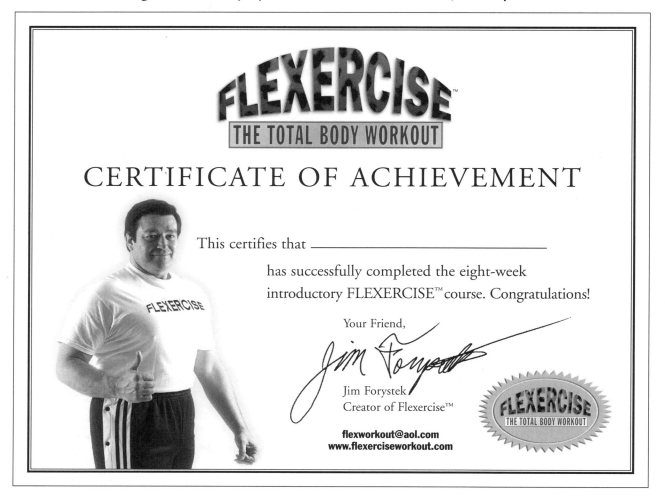

FLEXERCISE™
THE TOTAL BODY WORKOUT

CERTIFICATE OF ACHIEVEMENT

This certifies that _____

has successfully completed the eight-week
introductory FLEXERCISE™ course. Congratulations!

Your Friend,

Jim Forystek

Jim Forystek
Creator of Flexercise™

flexworkout@aol.com
www.flexerciseworkout.com

FLEXERCISE
THE TOTAL BODY WORKOUT

✂ -

Cut out and complete this application.

Mail this application to:
Please include a self-addressed stamped 9" x 12" envelope.

Flexercise™
2600 East 26th Street
Minneapolis, MN 55406

Name_____ **Age**_____

Address_____

State_____ **Zip Code**_____

I promise that I have successfully completed the eight-week introductory Flexercise™ course.

Signature_____